Get Your Zen On

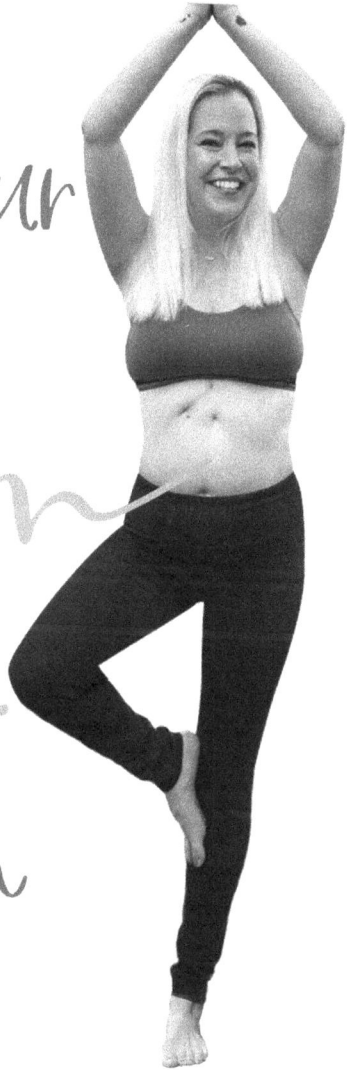

Kathleen Pope

Get Your Zen On

The book information is catalogued as follows;

Author Name(s): Kathleen Pope
Title:Get Your Zen On
Description: First Edition

1st Edition, 2021

Book Design by Lynda Mangoro

Edited by Lyndsay Fogarty

Photo credits: Tony Marotta (front cover), Trudi Derbyshire (back cover)

ISBN: 978-1-914447-07-5

ISBN (ebook): 978-1-914447-08-2

Prepared by That Guy's House Ltd.

www.ThatGuysHouse.com

Get Your Zen On

In this candid memoir and self-help guide, Zen Enthusiast Kathleen Pope invites you to travel with her on a journey of overcoming struggles and discovering inner strength.

Kathleen learned early on to not let anything break her spirit, starting with heart surgery when she was just five months old. Through the support of her mother, she was encouraged to believe in a beautiful future ahead and with great courage, she left her hometown in New Jersey and moved to Orlando to pursue a career at a world-famous theme park. Though she soon began to see her dreams coming true, Kathleen still faced many challenges but with the principles of God, Love, and Faith on her side, she developed the talent to find her Zen no matter what.

This emotional and uplifting guide encourages readers to celebrate life, find inner peace and ultimately Get Their Zen On.

Contents

Introduction

Merriam-Webster

ZEN (noun)

1 : a Japanese sect of Mahayana Buddhism that aims at enlightenment by direct intuition through meditation.

2 : a state of calm attentiveness in which one's actions are guided by intuition rather than by conscious effort.

> *"Quit hiding your magic!*
> *The world is ready for you!"*
> – Danielle Doby

I am just like you. I am trying to find my sense of Zen every day in this crazy, beautiful world. Some days are easier than others. Other days, I find it really challenging, and this was before COVID-19. These days are extra challenging in the new world of a pandemic. Through the years, I found the tools that help me, and I have shared these tools with friends and family. If you come along with me on this adventure, I will share them with you.

I do want to be open with you. I believe that vulnerability is power and strength, but it is a gift as well. There is so much we can learn from everyone, even if it is small. I believe that if you touch one life, you touch many. Our knowledge is passed on and on, person to person, through a brilliant ripple effect. "All you need is one mic." -Nas

If you can take anything positive or inspiring from my book and share it with just one person, we can change lives together. How exciting is that? The other day I read that privacy is power, but I also believe it is important to share our lives, too. People keep their lives private to protect themselves. I have been given permission from family and friends to share some very private stories. The stories of my family are most sacred and, until now, have been reserved only for our closest friends. All I ask is that you read the stories I share with compassion. Some of this was not easy to write, and I hesitated on the story that I will share about my dad.

The reason I am writing "Get Your Zen On" is because I am a work in progress, trying to achieve my Zen on a daily basis. I am still healing from past traumas and making mistakes daily. I am also experiencing success and inspiring people along the way.

I am blessed to have a tribe of friends. We encourage and uplift each other and, without them, I would be lost. Life is not meant to be lived alone. I am beyond thankful to the men and women in my life like, Marnie, Marie, Jody, Elaine, my mom, my sister, Judy (aka mom #2), my dad, my stepfather, Ken Walley, Jim, Valentina, Lisa, Clint, my "brother" Alex, Chef Tony, Nate, etc. I am blessed with too many to mention, so if I left you out, it was not on purpose. If you are in my life, you mean a lot to me.

At this point in my life, I have done about 15 years of research, asking my favorite question of strangers, coworkers, family and friends. What do you do for yourself? How do you relax? How do you balance your stress?

Now I ask you...

How do you *"Get Your Zen On?"*

I have battled anxiety and depression my whole life, so seeking happiness comes naturally. Finding happiness can be challenging at times. Some days I really get in my head. The biggest thing I ever did to fix the happiness in my outer world was to pack up my 1998 Dodge Durango in 2002 and move. I was 22 years old and moved from northern New Jersey down to Orlando, Florida.

Growing up, we were blessed to vacation in Orlando several times. My mother has always been a fan of what I will call the "World Dreams Theme Park." She is one of the biggest kids I know. We knew it as a magical place because of the energy felt walking through its streets. Just as the founder wanted, it is a place where you can leave all worries behind and just be. When you are in the parks, they are your world, and there is a sense of joy and excitement all around for all ages.

I did it! I ran to the dreamiest place on earth! This adventure was exciting and exhilarating. My goal was to get an apartment and a job at World Dreams Parks and Resorts. I was going to start a new life. I was running from any piece of unhappiness in New Jersey. It was a fresh start.

I achieved my goal and began a career with World Dreams almost immediately. Would you be surprised if I told you this didn't solve my inner world battles? The quick move was supposed to be a quick fix and a fresh start. Lack of planning brought repercussions, such as financial difficulty, which was overwhelming for years.

Now, as much as wisdom comes with age, there is still a lot to learn. In this book, I will be sharing my mistakes in the hope that you can learn from them and maybe avoid some suffering. I believe our time on this planet is meant for growing and learning as much as possible. This can be beautiful and painful. Nothing I share with you is new; it is simply my story. You all have your stories, too - different experiences but the same lessons and the same truths. I hope my story resonates with you. These lessons are ancient. You fall down and you get back up. Some call it "the game of life."

When I signed my publishing contract in 2017, it was a dream come true. I was excited to share parts of my story! I was and still am hoping to inspire, encourage, motivate, and entertain those who want to take a glimpse into my personal journey. I had found the right publisher, and he had found me. We were on the same page immediately with the vision I had for my book and the impact I wanted to have. I thought people may be interested in and be moved to try some of the methods I have used to bring myself back up when life's lessons got me down. I hope you will be.

On a daily basis, I am still being tested on my principals and notice rewards when I succeed. Like you, I live, I learn, and I never stop learning. "The teacher is the student, and the student is the teacher," as they say.

Life is definitely the biggest professor. They say the universe will test you until you get it right, including revisiting lessons you still need that you thought you were through. I find this to be very accurate.

I still consider myself a Jersey girl living in Florida. My entire family is still in New Jersey and New York. My Jersey pride is strong but so is my Orlando pride. In 2016, after the Pulse Nightclub shooting, it was amazing to see and be a part of Orlando uniting.

I am proud of the work I did for World Dreams. I am proud that I was brave enough to move down here by myself. I have only called my parents 100 times to beg them to let me move back home. Yes, seriously. My mother always reminded me of how much I accomplished in Florida and how I really liked the life I made for myself down here. I don't have blood family down here, but I chose a family down here. My friends have supported me through the good and the bad, and I think I can say that I have done the same. It is f***ing hard adulting. It looks so much better in the movies and on TV.

> *"Life is truly a dance between the inner and outer - a journey of your human needs and soul desires."*
>
> – Unknown

Life doesn't come with an instruction manual, so the more we share, the more we learn. Sometimes the best thing we can learn or are reminded of is that we are not alone. YOU are not alone.

We are not only the teacher, but we are the students. In all reality, we are all messengers. We all have the power to share a message of hope or despair. I have personally found that life is like a rollercoaster, and I remind myself of that when I am down. It is just a matter of time until God, the universe, and angels guide and lift me up. I am spiritual but not religious, but we will get to that later. You will find out I don't like labels. I would rather remain outside the box, open to all opportunities and discoveries.

I hope you are inspired by what you read and share what works for you with others. Like they say, everyone is fighting a battle we know nothing about, so be kind. This includes being kind to yourself. It is never too late to learn how to love yourself. It took me a while, and some days, I don't like myself, my thoughts, or my actions. I am still learning, still growing, and still practicing every day. So, I focus on the small victories - and the big ones, too - looking at how far I have come.

Don't expect your healing to happen overnight or by a particular age or time. I am still healing and in search of a new way to find Zen every day. If there is one thing my journey has taught me, it is that I do not know everything. I will never know everything. No one does. I have found that approaching most things as a novice is a great tool. We can learn something new every day if we leave our egos at the door and keep an open mind.

I hope you can learn from my mistakes. I hope I can help you find Zen on your average days, greatest days, and shitty days too. Just as all other authors, I am more of a guide or a companion on your journey than anything. This is where I sincerely thank you for allowing me to be part of your life. I also want to welcome you to mine.

The Move

I was having suicidal thoughts in 2002. On paper, I had EVERYTHING. I had an on-and-off boyfriend with status. I was a successful manager of two boutiques in Bergen County, New Jersey. I was majoring in business at Ramapo College, and I had an apartment in Wyckoff, a very status-driven and prestigious town. Think: "Real Housewives of New Jersey." They literally film those ladies in that town. I never had money like that, but that is what I grew up around. I knew it was achievable and it was what I wanted. I wanted that success and status. Most days, I was motivated. I would drive to work in my red convertible Mustang, singing along to the music I was playing like everything was great. Sunny days with the top down were my Zen.

I was managing two Feng Shui boutiques. One boutique was in Ridgewood, New Jersey, and one was in Midland Park, New Jersey. Both towns are upper middle class to upper class. The stores were owned by one woman only: my mentor, Elaine. She would come to have one of the biggest influences on my life. She is a very special lady with special gifts and beauty inside and out.

There is a lot of money and influence circling areas like Ridgewood. Celebrities, high-powered attorneys, successful business owners, and more frequented both shops. At the time, Feng Shui was bigger in New York and California, though it was beginning to catch on locally. I think a lot of people saw the ancient art of Feng Shui as trendy.

Ridgewood, New Jersey is a beautiful little town that neighbors the town where I grew up. The streets in the heart of town are laced with mom and pop coffee shops, boutiques and a fancy, well-known chain coffee shop. There are award-winning salons, and every restaurant makes a great date spot with delicious food and atmosphere. Day and night, people walk the main street up and down, from the movie theater to the town's oldest coffee shop. They shop or window shop while enjoying the scenery and relaxing in this close-knit community.

Bookends is the town's exclusive bookstore, known for hosting book signings by celebrity authors. I was able to meet the extraordinary Deepak Chopra there. It was exhilarating. That's right, I have met Deepak Chopra.

Deepak Chopra is an Indian-American author who is an advocate for alternative medicine. In the new age movement, he is a prominent figure. His books, videos, and recorded audio meditations have made him one of the best-known advocates in the world. Before coming to the United States in 1970, Deepak studied medicine in India. He met Maharishi Mahesh Yogi, an Indian guru, in 1985, and he became involved in the Transcendental Movement, also known as TM. The program is an advanced meditation practice with millions of followers seeking world peace. This is a wonderful movement, and you may be interested in doing more research on this.

Deepak gained his following after being a guest on the Oprah Winfrey show. He was a physician in India and when he first entered the states. His occupation shifted with his study of the mind-body connection. In 1996, Deepak co-founded the Chopra Center for Wellbeing. He is someone I continue to follow and highly respect. He has paved the way for many on the path to alternative healing.

I was enjoying the town of Ridgewood on a sunny, summer afternoon, and while I was having lunch and shopping, I stumbled across Elaine and her Feng Shui boutique. I did not know it was a Feng Shui boutique or even what Feng Shui was. It was called The Purple Pear, and the name was enough to draw me in.

Upon entering the shop, I was comforted by the intoxicating atmosphere. The smell of incense was enchanting, as was the decor. I recognized Buddha statues, and there were a lot of new figure statues that I was totally intrigued by but had no idea what they represented. Three-legged frog statues, King Kun, Kwan Yin, and others surrounded me with their unique powers.

I was fascinated and felt connected. I felt comforted in this space. I was literally in a room with Zen gardens, books on Zen, and books on the mind-body connection. I had always believed in self-healing, and this store was my introduction to learning that it was true for many.

Journal Prompt

Write about a moment you experienced through your body and senses as a feeling of being "home" in a new place.

_____

_____

_____

_____

_____

Elaine was a kindred spirit. The Purple Pear became my second home and changed my life forever. It was a new chapter of my journey that I am still living today. Elaine had, and still has, so much education and wisdom to offer the world. She studies Feng Shui, Chinese Astrology, Numerology, etc. She is also psychic.

Originating from ancient China, Feng Shui uses energy forces to find harmony in different spaces. You can use it in your home, office, garden, and more. In English, the words "Feng Shui" literally translate into "wind-water." Using the space around you, it is possible to attract good health, wealth, money, and love.

My relationship with Elaine was special, and her guidance and encouragement into a new realm was important. I knew this had existed, but I could not find it. My intuition and empathy became heightened. I increased my prayers. I prayed to God, angels and Jesus for guidance and resources and, of course, protection. Again, I am not religious, only spiritual.

I plunged into this new knowledge. I discovered books such as "The Four

Agreements" on the bookshelves at the store. To this day, I believe if the 4 agreements were read and taught in schools today, this simple act would change the world. If you ask me, it is a must read. I always keep 2 copies of this book on my shelf. One is mine and the second is to give away when the moment presents itself.

It goes like this...

1. Be impeccable with your word.

2. Don't take anything personally.

3. Don't make assumptions.

4. Always do your best.

It seems simple doesn't it? Read the book and try to practice every day. That's right, practice.

I became intrigued and had more interest in becoming a Feng Shui consultant than I did in my business degree at Ramapo College, where my parents were paying my tuition. This caused friction between my parents and me. My family is great, and they are the most important people in my life; however, in 2002, we were disagreeing over decisions I was making regarding career choices and my education. They wanted me to put my studies first over the store.

I wasn't happy. I was somewhat aware that I had depression and anxiety, but back in that day, mental health was not talked about. It wasn't normal to be on medication. It wasn't viewed as taking care of yourself. People like me had a big stigma.

When my boyfriend and I would argue, it was not unlike him to call me crazy. It hurt. I knew I wasn't perfect. I had a chemical imbalance, and it wasn't my fault. I wanted help. I did get some. I saw a psychiatrist and was put on a couple meds. They worked, I guess, or they didn't. I am a very emotional woman and crying and screaming at my boyfriend was not unlike me. In my defense, he was not the right man for me. He was cheating. I should have followed my intuition and found the strength to let him go. We were young, although I thought 19 and 21 were mature ages.

Looking back, thank goodness he didn't want to get married at that age. He knew back then that he didn't want to get married until he was 30. How funny. How wise. I wish I had enjoyed my youth more being single than in relationships. I used to think I wanted to get married and have babies by age 25 or 26.

Jake had a strong pull on me. I believed he was my soul mate. I always have believed and now, more than ever, I believe in multiple soul mates. He is one for sure. He had a big impact on my life. I was able to love him unconditionally. He was my first intimate relationship, so our bond was really strong, at least for me because I gave him all of me.

In recent years, we reconnected, and he apologized for his behavior and the way he treated me. I was able to forgive him. We were both so young, and he was wise enough to know that settling down and getting married at 19 and 21 was not the right road for us to travel. For me, it was heartbreaking. I saw him as my present and future back when we were those kids. We had broken up several times before, but our final break up was the most painful. This influenced my decision to move to Florida.

One day, I went to my boss Elaine, who was more than a mentor. She had become like a mother to me, guiding and teaching me in so many ways. I told her how unhappy I was and that I didn't want to be around anymore. She knew what I meant and said that wasn't an option.

She asked me, if I were to move and start over, where would I want to go? I told her California or Florida with World Dreams Parks in mind. She said I wasn't ready for California. It was too hard for me and I was too soft. She then asked me where I wanted to go in Florida and, without hesitation, I replied, "Orlando. I want to work at World Dreams."

Elaine advised me that is where I should go. Within days, I was packing up my 1998 Dodge Durango. My boss had given me money like a severance package. Her advice was to leave Friday, when our conversation had only taken place that Monday. She said that if I were to think about things too long, I would change my mind on the move. Elaine was probably right.

I remember visiting my mom the day I was leaving. It is very hard to look back on and still makes me tear up to this day. She gave me some money and a laptop. It had always been my dream to write a book. She cried and, thinking about it now, I could cry. I remember mom's embrace. It was surreal to us both. Looking back on it now, I wish I had never left. Leaving my family makes me sad to this day. That is why I am keeping this brief for now. There are several times in Florida that I have regretted my move, but I have also made a pretty good life down here and have had much success. I have met so many wonderful people that I consider extended family.

I left New Jersey with my resume and some money and drove down to Florida. It was a beautiful drive. The leaves on the trees were magnificent colors as I was driving in early November. The Carolinas were the best. I drove 8 hours a day for 3 days. Every night, I got a good night's sleep at a hotel. I was not lonely. I was excited. I was so adventurous back in those days; I believed anything was possible and that the move would be so easy.

Upon landing in Orlando, I settled at a hotel across the street from a famous Orlando theme park known for its Hollywood-style rides and attractions. I started to hunt for an apartment and a job immediately. I didn't realize it would be hard to get a job without having an apartment first and hard to get an apartment without proof of income. It was difficult changing banks, and my car insurance went up because there are more uninsured drivers in the Orlando area.

I spent my first Floridian Thanksgiving in that hotel across from the theme park, happily eating the best rotisserie chicken restaurant's Holiday Turkey special. I love that rotisserie chicken chain restaurant. I was not lonely. I was so excited. I was practically on vacation. Most days were extraordinarily sunny. Everywhere I went there were palm trees. There was always a reminder that I was in Florida. I had really done it. I had left New Jersey. I had no idea what I had gotten myself into.

Journal Prompt

What is the bravest thing you've ever done? What would you tell your past self now?

_____

_____

_____

_____

_____

So, the moral of the story is plan, plan, plan! It is great to be spontaneous, but with something as big as moving out of state to start over, plan a little. If I had come down here with a clear plan, I would not have struggled so much. If I had prepared and researched the area for apartments, I would have spent less time living in a pricey hotel. If I knew the balance between Florida's pay scale and New Jersey's, I would not have been shocked that my first job in Florida at the Millenia mall started me at $7.50. At the time in Orlando, this was not a bad retail starting rate; however, this would not provide enough to pay my bills, and that ultimately would be the beginning of my financial downfall.

I had my own one-bedroom, 725-square-foot apartment in Kissimmee, Florida (close to World Dreams), a car payment, insurance, etc. I was scared about how I was going to pay my bills. I racked my credit cards up and missed payments on other bills. I didn't know what to do, so I thought, "Let me try waitressing."

I knew waiters and waitresses worked for tips and could make pretty good money. I called my mom with this idea. She said there was no way I could be a waitress because I am too tiny. I am only 4' 10", though sometimes I say I am 4' 11". Although it has not always been easy, I certainly proved her wrong. I excelled as a server and fell in love with the restaurant business. That did not come easy either.

I didn't have any restaurant experience. All my experience was in retail. So, no one would hire me. I immediately thought about a popular American fare, Irish hospitality restaurant. It was the place to go and the place to work. I applied at least three times, but they refused to hire me due to lack of experience. I really wanted to work there! This is funny because I have made serving (or waitressing) my career. At the time, it was not funny; it was disappointing.

The first restaurant to hire me was a popular casual dining chain restaurant. It was a great company, and I am thankful to this day for the opportunity they gave me. It was a fun job, and I learned a lot. It is where I got my experience to go to Dreams. You had to have at least 2 years of experience to even apply to work at Dreams as a server.

Today, it is even harder to get into than it was back then, and it was never easy. Dreams has approximately 75,000 employees in Orlando, Lake Buena Vista, and Celebration. It is competitive. When I applied, it was before people would apply online. I went directly to the World Dreams HR building, where they still hold interviews today. The HR building is cute and, without giving too much away, it is totally themed out.

I had 2 years of experience, great references and a referral from a girlfriend who was a lifeguard coordinator at World Dreams Tropical water park. I was so excited. I was thrilled. I started at World Dreams Nautical Resort at a moderate restaurant at the high-end resort. It was there that I met a mentor and friend, Chef Tony Marotta, and a dear friend, Steve Sapiro, both of whom I am very close with today. So much so, I have not changed their names in this book.

There are many other long-lasting relationships that I have made over the years through working at World Dreams Parks and Resorts. I have met some amazing people at Dreams and, of course, like anywhere else, some not so great. I try to focus on the positive relationships that I made. I know that both good and bad experiences helped me to grow personally and professionally.

Journal Prompt

Name at least two people who have significantly inspired your personal and professional growth.

_____

_____

_____

_____

_____

The Dreamiest

It did not take long in my career at World Dreams to discover that Dreams was not the dreamiest place for me. It is a beautiful and magical place but, just like other parts of the world, behind the scenes is another story entirely. Many coworkers, or team members, are suffering through life while "making dreams come true" for families, couples and singles. These people are the magic. They come in to work and give the guest an experience like no other. I know many of you can relate in your own work areas and careers.

The truth is that while they are providing the world with smiles and magic, they may have personal struggles that no one knows about. Some of these team members are even homeless. Dreams Park pays so little to their hourly staff. It is so easy to say, "Go get another job," or "Go get a better education." Where is the advancement opportunity for these men and women? As many of you know, it is very hard to advance at such a large company.

I believe when you work years for a company and dedicate yourself, you should be taken care of and given the opportunity to advance. That should be the company's responsibility and goal for their long-time employees. People working for companies earning billions of dollars should not be struggling to make ends meet and having to work 2 to 3 jobs. I am sure many of you are experiencing similar situations and must work 2 to 3 jobs in this economy.

I was in a different department and a different role. Dreams Park was not paying me - their guests were. As a bartender and a server, I was tipped. I was blessed. My salary was dependent upon our guests, and most of them really took care of us. That did not make me stop caring about my coworkers who were hourly, just trying to make a better life for themselves.

We all experience pain, loss, and tragedy, and, just like the rest of the world, at Dreams we keep on working 365 days of the year, 24 hours a day and 7 days a week. The difference is that while we are hurting inside, we still bring a smile to our guests and help them celebrate their special times. There are plenty who fight depression and anxiety on a daily basis while at work and also many other obstacles that our closest friends don't even know about. These people are so brave to me. There is also great joy found working at Dreams. For many, working at Dreams could be an escape from having to face our real lives.

I think it is impossible not to smile watching children in awe of the magic around them. In a land of fantasy and happiness, nothing is impossible. They are brought into a world they believe to be real and, to them, it is. Meeting a princess is a dream come true, while seeing a villain might be a little scary. The rides are more than special and uplifting. Individuals of all ages can enjoy them. Watching through a child's eyes is a gift to us all. This kind of experience reminds you of a simpler time and that dreams still exist. There is hope and magic left in this world for those who believe.

On days I was not feeling my best, I would simply talk to any child and ask them about their day. Hearing these little ones so excited to meet their favorite characters, see a castle or ride their favorite rides always reminded me that I was incredibly blessed to be doing my job and living where people vacation. I would look outside to the sun, crystal clear skies, and palm trees. I worked at a place where families saved for years to visit. Dreams really do come true at World Dreams Parks and Resorts. The opportunities I had at that workplace are like no other, and I will share many of those stories later. I am also so grateful for all the opportunities the company provided me. Who else would let me sing on stage with American country singer and actor Trace Adkins? Ask my mom, I don't have a professional singing voice!

Working for World Dreams was my destiny. The passion I had working there was great. I was a trainer, I taught classes, and I was cross-trained to bartend, host, and facilitate classes outside my role as a server. I really don't believe that servers grow up desiring to make serving a career. I watched and listened, discovering that the long-term, full-time servers and bartenders in the exclusive restaurants were making between $80,000 to $100,000 a year, even back in 2004. This is one of the major reasons I wanted to make serving my full-time career. As a young, part time server, I knew it would take a lot of time but would be worth it.

Journal Prompt

What are your favorite things to do? What brings you joy and Zen? How do you incorporate them into your work?

_____

_____

_____

_____

_____

"A dream is a wish your heart makes."

-Lily James

Dreams is a seniority-based company. That is a positive and negative thing. Your education and skill is pushed to the side as someone with less skill or less education gets a full-time position over you simply because they have been with the company longer.

The longing was there, and I fantasized about being a full-time server in the parks, making six figures a year. I could get a similar full-time position with the company if I just held out for 20 years, so it was achievable. There is a saying within the company that us hopefuls pass along: "'Full-time servers with seniority have to die or retire for you to get their spot."

We all know it. Full-timers easily have 30 years seniority. It is not unlikely for your server at a World Dreams restaurant to be around 60 years old. My passion for World Dreams Park exceeded my expectations for the career I was looking to achieve within the company.

Through social media and keeping in touch with my friends back home, I envied their career choices and success. Some of my friends envied mine. It didn't matter what I did for World Dreams, just the fact that I worked for them had a status. The company is well-known for their high standards and being selective on who they hire. Working for World Dream' stands out on any resume, no matter what title you hold.

I wasn't making that much money. I was living more like paycheck to paycheck, to be honest. The restaurant I was working in was not busy. I was at the deluxe World Dreams Nautical Resort, yet I was at a moderate restaurant. I did not work at the Nautical Resort's steakhouse, but I did host there a couple times through some of my cross-training. I was blessed to be cross-trained for bartending at the lounge. Guests could get a drink while waiting for their table. You didn't have to eat at the steakhouse to enjoy the lounge. Anyone could come in for drinks and a snack. It was a popular place to be.

I found that being an adult still came with a lot of bills, and I was forced to have a second job during my entire part-time career at World Dreams. I did not leave my casual dining restaurant chain when I got my part-time job with World Dreams. This was a smart move, as it provided extra income and a new lesson in life. My lesson was David, my fiancé.

"I knew it from the start, you would break my heart...
but still I had to play this painful part."

-Milli Vanilli

David and I worked at the casual dining chain restaurant together. When we met, I had a boyfriend, and it was almost a year later that David and I would begin dating. He was a manager of mine. It started very innocently; in fact, I had no idea that he was interested. He asked me on a secret date. He was not allowed to date the staff and, to my knowledge, he hadn't. We started seeing each other and there was an immediate connection. I really liked him, and he was good to me. We didn't hop into bed. He was very patient as I made him wait until I was comfortable.

We dated for a year before we became engaged. He was a good man; we were just really young. I was 25 and he was 26. I didn't know at the time, but I was not ready for marriage. David was pretty successful, climbing the ranks at our chain restaurant into management. He continued to get promotions and his own store. I had left the company when we moved in together.

I spent more time at World Dreams. Even on my days off, I was on World Dreams' property, taking courses at Dreams College, which is located behind the scenes. Tons of courses are offered there along with mandatory classes that we all took to be a team member. World Dreams College is not an accredited institution; however, the courses offered are delivered by experienced professionals. You must work there to enroll in any of the courses. Dreams College provides instructor-led classroom sessions and seminars as well as online learning. I took advantage of every opportunity. I have always loved learning and ongoing education. These courses were expanding my resume, which I was determined to expand in case the server dream didn't come true.

I was offered the food and beverage coordinator position at Dreams Tropical Water Park in 2006. Although it was a low-paid, hourly position, it was still the beginning of my real advancement at the company. Before the coordinator position, I had facilitated multiple classes and trained at Dreams Nautical Resort. I was able to do the extra work assignments while still in the role of a part-time server. The coordinator position came with a new role, and for the first time, I was full-time with the company. However, being in a different role made it even harder to get a full-time position as a server. My full-time role as a food and beverage coordinator was only a tiny hourly rate, yet it came with a title. At age 25/26, I was really trying to move forward with the company that mattered to me.

My relationship with David suffered due to the competition that I had created between us. The more successful he was, the more successful I wanted to be. The time I invested in Dreams took away time from us. He hated the fact that even on my days off I was on the property. His feelings were justified. Being occupied at work for 7 days a week left little time for us.

We tried to make it work. David began saving for a house. We both wanted to get married and have a family. I didn't really get a chance to plan my wedding. We weren't in a huge rush; we picked 07/07/2007 as our date. We got engaged in October of 2005 on his birthday. By early 2006, things were really going downhill between us. The fights were getting hotter, and there were times that I took off my ring, which I then would keep in our jewelry box. Some of my friends at work knew what was going on. One day, I would be wearing my ring and the next day I wouldn't.

There were other things, too. David would accuse me of being jealous. There was a young hostess at his job, a 17-year-old kid. I knew she was interested in him by the stories he would tell about how she maximized their time at work together. Often, she would sit in his office crying to him about her personal problems at home. He assured me that he was just trying to be helpful. She turned 18, and he made her a server. She still would spend days in his office crying over her father mistreating her.

I had enough and ended up moving out to give us space. David urged me to go to couples counseling. I do believe that things are meant to be; however, I do regret not going to couples counseling with him. I was so stubborn and was really starting to give up. My idea was, why go to couple's counseling if we couldn't even live together? It wasn't long before his interest in me shifted to the girl he worked with. I don't have to tell you the rest of the story. She got pregnant, which caused a lot of heartache between both of us. Our life together, and our chapter, was finished - whether we wanted it to be or not.

I was devastated when David and I broke up. I threw myself into the coordinator role at Dreams, working 60 hours a week. It didn't help. I think it created more stress. I know it did. It was one of those times in Florida when I called my mom and asked her if I could come home. She didn't want me to move back. She didn't want me to run from what happened, but I needed a break. We agreed that I would come up for a couple weeks. I quit Dreams, as I needed to reevaluate everything in my life. What did I want in life? I had wanted a husband and children, but for now, that was off the table. I wanted World Dreams, but not the position I was in as a food and beverage coordinator.

I packed a couple bags, just enough to get me through a couple weeks knowing I could borrow or buy anything else that I needed while I was up in New Jersey. My goal was to move back home. A few friends knew I was coming up but not many. I usually keep my visits up north pretty quiet until I arrive. The reason I have always done this, and continue to do so, especially with my shorter trips, is because I prefer to spend as much time with my family as possible. I love my friends and seeing them, but my family is everything to me and, since I live out of state, I love to spend every moment with them. If my friends want to meet up, I invite them to visit my parents' house. My brother and sister take me out as well, and I will extend invitations to friends as another meet-up opportunity. Often, we will have one night out at a bar or a club just as a fun night for us.

My visit was great. My family went to work during the day, and I had a lot of time to relax by the lake and play on social media. My family still lives on the lake that I grew up on. We spent many summers swimming, fishing, and canoeing. In the winter, we would ice skate. Across the lake was a private beach. Each summer, we would get a membership there. Most families in the neighborhood there would do the same. I had my circle of summer friends that I would enjoy the lake with. Sometimes we would swim from the beach to my house and hang out there.

I caught up on my reading. The best part of being home is the home-cooked meals. My dad (stepfather) can really cook, and mom can really bake. We love dining out and seeing movies together. We visit the local bowling alley for some pin dropping and pool. My mother is really good at pool. We don't let her win, and she always kicks ass whether she is playing us or friends.

My dad is a Marine. My biological dad was in the Army. My mother is a military wife, and I was born at Fort Bragg, a military base in Fayetteville, North Carolina. Ok, I was born in a hospital, and we spent my early years on the base. I do have some early childhood memories of being raised there, but I don't have many memories of my parents being together, as they got divorced when I was younger. Before they got divorced, we moved to Massachusetts, where my father was stationed. That is where my sister was born.

My sister is a tough cookie. She will give you the shirt off her back and is the best woman I know on earth, but she is tough as nails. Colleen tells it like it is. She is blunt and she is honest, and she doesn't make excuses.

So, while I was in New Jersey trying to decide what to do without David, my family comforted me with tough love. They had loved David, as he spent a Christmas with us and asked my parents' permission to marry me before our engagement. Like I said, he was a good guy. I have forgiven him for everything. We were kids, and kids make mistakes. My family's advice was to move on because it was over. I wish I could have done that easily. I was only 26 and had so much time ahead of me, but I did not realize it back then. I had plenty of time to meet someone and have children. Fortunately, I also had the time to take a moment to heal. I needed time to heal. I had planned a life with David, and now I had to accept that was not going to happen.

It was a great time being up there in New Jersey, and it went really fast. I didn't want to leave, and I didn't want to return to Florida. I had no plan for what I was going to do or even what I wanted to do. My heart was still broken. I swear to this day that the emotional pain of a heartbreak takes longer to heal from then heart surgery, and I would know as I have had four. To find my Zen during this time I read, prayed, spoke to friends, drank too much, and listened to a lot of music. The songs I played were happy and sad. I did a lot of crying, which I believe is super healing. I believe after a good cry you can really feel a release. That peace is certainly Zen.

After visiting my family in New Jersey, I made my way to Manassas, Virginia, 45 minutes outside of Washington D.C. My biological father lives there with my stepmother, Natasha. My parents divorced when my sister and I were young. I was about 6 years old, and my sister was about 3. I spent time with him and Natasha in a similar way. We went to the museums and the Kennedy Center, and my stepmother cooked for us.

My stepmother is Russian, and even if we eat out, she always puts out fresh snacks, cookies, and juice. We went to the movie theater and even an international movie theater. I remember seeing "Little Miss Sunshine" - what a great movie. We went out to dinner and frequented a cute little coffee shop called Cafe Mozart. If you get a chance to go there, I recommend it.

We talked about David, and my dad's advice was to take the time to heal. This time with them really brought me Zen. We drank tea and spoke openly about trying to get a plan together. I did tell my father I wanted to move back to New Jersey. I let him know that my mother was against it, as she didn't want me to run home. She really believed that I would be happier in Florida. He agreed.

Journal Prompt

"Sometimes things need to break so that we can fix them." What is not working in your life right now? If you were to release or break free from it, how would that bring you more Zen?

_____

_____

_____

_____

_____

"Release past pain or it will slow you down."

-Unknown

I didn't have so much money that I could just continue to travel and heal, so I made my way back to Orlando and stayed with some gracious friends. I moved in temporarily with a couple that was mutual friends of David and me. They knew how much I was hurting and really wanted to see me happy again. They were kind and compassionate. They would cook for me and start my mornings off by handing me a cup of fresh coffee and encouraging me to keep going. I got a part-time job serving at a local restaurant and started my plan to rebuild my life in Florida.

Serving jobs outside of the Orlando theme parks are different in a few ways, but perhaps the biggest way they are different is the money. On theme park properties, you make good money and consistent money. Theme parks have consistent traffic and people come from all over the world for these experiences, but we also have our regular locals. The restaurants at the parks are award-winning, so locals and travelers alike enjoy a breakfast, lunch, or dinner on a night out.

I needed to at least get back to a bigger company, even if it was outside the parks, so I left the local restaurant. I began serving at Caribbean's Soft Wind, a well-known restaurant down here and one of my favorites. The food and the atmosphere are so good. Caribbean's Soft Wind is a chain restaurant and a great company to work for. This chain is part of a very successful company with an array of famous restaurants.

If I had been working at an upscale restaurant or working in downtown Orlando, I would have made more money. At the time, I didn't have the experience for an upscale restaurant, and I was not too close to downtown Orlando and did not have the most reliable transportation.

"Time does not heal all wounds, we do."

-Unknown

Once I was back on my feet, I moved in with another good friend named Taylor. Taylor and I met back in 2004 at the Nautical Resort where we worked with Chef Tony and our friend, Steve. She was no longer with the Dreams company either. She was living 40 minutes away and attending the University of Central Florida. As fate would have it, we crossed paths again working at Caribbean Soft Wind.

Taylor is one of my favorite people to this day. She is hardworking, spontaneous, and loves to travel. She is the one who got me into online dating. I was never interested in online dating, but her words still echo in my head: "Why limit yourself on who you can meet?"

Online dating has been interesting and really kind of fun. I have actually made a couple of friends through the sites. There were a few occasions where there was no spark between my date and me, but we both mutually liked each other as people. One of the men I met years ago was Calvin, a lawyer. I met Calvin through a well-known dating website, and as a lawyer, he will look over contracts for me and answer questions for free. He is a good friend and a great lawyer, so for me, I get a bonus. Calvin is handsome and looks like Jim Caviezel. He has a great personality. Today, he still tells stories of his dates, which sometimes are very funny, and we laugh hard together.

As happy as I was at work and at home with Taylor and friends, I was still recovering from my heartbreak. I knew David's new girlfriend was pregnant, so of course I thought about that. His betrayal had caught me off guard. I had promised to spend my life with this man. So, I had to concentrate on myself and "Get My Zen On." Taylor was a fun girl. She kept me busy. We had wine, movie, vision board, and game nights. She was not a girl to ever sit around sad, and she wasn't going to let me do that either. I love you Taylor!

Taylor and I lived in the Winter Springs area, about 20 minutes outside Orlando. Winter Springs is a nice area and close to UCF. We lived in a house owned by a man that had graduated from UCF. He was in his 20s; we all were. His parents had helped him purchase the three-bedroom property, and he rented out the two spare bedrooms. One was open when I reunited with Taylor and she knew I was looking for a place. I met her landlord/roommate, and it was a done deal.

I have fond memories of the three of us living together. I went through some hard times there too, but Taylor and I were there for each other and it really helped. Along with still getting over David, Taylor helped me start dating again. Work was good but I wasn't making that much money. I was living paycheck to paycheck and I had some car trouble and was without a car until I could afford to fix it. This was a few months where I relied on friends for transportation.

During my time living with Taylor, I also was bitten on the neck by a brown recluse spider. Let me tell you about the brown recluse spider. It is native to the United States, from Texas to Florida. In North America, the brown recluse is one of three spiders with medically significant venom. The spider's necrotic venom produces a flesh-eating disease, and it started to create a hole in my neck.

I had not known I had been bit at the time and thought I was having some strange acne, as it started out looking like a painful zit. It got to a stage where it was too large and so painful that I couldn't sleep. I tried to pop it. TMI for you? Anyway, as it grew larger, I realized it was eating my skin. I went to my general care physician, but the antibiotics she prescribed did not help. I ended up in the emergency room, where they were able to do a procedure where they cut a hole in my neck, scraped the poison out and then packed it with an antibacterial gauze. I had to take stronger antibiotics and have the packing removed two or three days later. I survived and I hate spiders.

Journal Prompt

High Vibe Home: What are 10 things in your home or about your home that bring you Zen?

_____

_____

_____

_____

_____

"Your Life Unfolds In Proportion To Your Courage."
–Danielle LaPorte

I lived in the Winter Springs area for over a year. Of course, it was my plan to return to Orlando and work for Dreams again. My best friend Jenny (who also worked with Taylor, Steve, Chef Tony and I at Dreams) asked me to move in with her. Jenny was still with the Dreams company. All of my friends were asking me to come back, especially Jenny.

We shopped for a two-bedroom apartment in Orlando. Our ideal place was a nice commute to Dreams property. My friend Tommy was able to get us a great deal in a resort-style apartment within walking distance to the Millenia Mall. Ah, the Millenia Mall. The Millenia Mall in Orlando is one of the most popular places for locals and tourists. It consists of high-end stores and great restaurants.

Jenny helped me get back to Dreams. She encouraged me to go on my interview. I was hired back as a bartender, but they were on a hiring freeze so I would have to wait a bit for them to place me at a particular location. I knew it was a part-time bartending position, and over the years, I often worked two jobs like so many other team members.

I was able to get a job at the Famous Cheesecake in Orlando, located inside the Millenia Mall.

Ok, actually the Famous Cheesecake that I was hired at and got my experience at was in Winter Park, Florida, about 20-25 minutes from our apartment. That was the one hiring at the time. After working there for several months, I was able to transfer to the one at the Millenia mall.

Between the locals and tourists, this is one of the busiest Famous Cheesecakes in the United States. Like Caribbean Soft Wind, this job was great, with super nice staff, and I still have friends from there today. The company is great to work for. The price point was higher, so the tips were better, except for the assholes that didn't tip. If you are in the business, you know the groups I am talking about. There are certain groups, such as foreigners, that don't tip because the country they come from doesn't tip their servers. They are not the only ones, unfortunately. Tip your servers. We work hard and provide you your experience. You can eat at home; you dine out for an experience.

During my time at the Famous Cheesecake, I met a very special man named Sean (okay, I changed his name here). Sean was a bartender, and I was a server. We had minimal interaction, as I collected the drinks that he made for my tables. We also saw each other at store meetings. He was funny and social with a lot of the servers; I just wasn't one of them.

Sean was a very hard-working man, very balanced and seemed responsible, especially as he became a single father. Sean had a child and a girlfriend when I met him. They split up and Sean became the primary caretaker of Eva (her name has also been changed). Sean was all about his daughter. He still is. He is a great dad, and he has always been hands-on with everything, from changing diapers to teaching his daughter the alphabet song.

I had worked with Sean for a year before he asked me out. I found him attractive, probably since the first day I saw him. As I spoke with him, his personality was even more attractive. He had a great sense of humor and was very funny. He had an easy time making me laugh. Our small interactions became like a dance of flirtation. I was single at the time, and he definitely had my interest.

I still remember the day he asked me out. I didn't know if he was serious. He was done bartending for the day and was collecting tips from servers. As servers, we tipped our bartenders for the service they provided us by making the drinks for our tables. I was standing right by him, ready to give my tip. He said, "Ms. Pope, do you like Italian food?"

I smiled and said, "Yes I do."

He pretended to make a note of it on the paper he was holding. It was adorable. It was close to Christmas, so we agreed to wait until New Year's was over to go out. Neither of us dated people from work, and those were our reputations at the Famous Cheesecake. We were in our 30s and knew it wasn't always a good idea to blend work with romance. The holidays came and went, and the flirting continued, but he was yet to formally set a date for our date.

One day, I just went up to Sean at the bar when the restaurant was closed and no one was around. I told Sean that I was older, and I understood that he and his daughter were a package deal. I told him that I worked at World Dreams and we could go there on a date with her. I did not mind if she was part of our date at all. I wanted to get to know this sweet man outside of work. He asked me to go out with him that night. That very night was our first date. Eva was with her mother's parents.

We went to a Mexican restaurant called Grandpa's Mexican. Our conversation was great. There was a connection, and he was a gentleman, walking me to my car, but he did not kiss me. We kept up our flirtation at work and went out again and again. I met his friends and his daughter, and within two weeks we were official. Again, we had known each other a year, so it didn't feel like we were jumping into things. It felt right. I can look back today and still know that I made a great decision, even if we rushed in after only two weeks of dating. Usually rushing doesn't work out, but this was an exception to the rule. This would have no impact on our breakup. That was for different reasons.

"Your life is not going to crumble if you allow yourself to be vulnerable."

-Me (Kathleen)

The first time that I met Eva, she was shy. I had gone over to Sean's house, and it was close to her bedtime. She was the cutest little thing ever. She had on her pink princess nightie and was carrying her sippy cup. She was a year and 9 months old. She had curly blonde hair and Sean had nicknamed her "Curly."

As mine and Sean's relationship progressed, I spent more and more time with her. I was her "Kafween." Eva had angelic hugs and a contagious smile. She was smart and loved to play. We had tea parties and played hide and go seek often. Dolls and tents were part of our routine, too. We became best buddies. Sean called us two peas in a pod. I never imagined how meeting them would change my life forever. I carry fond memories of our time together to this day, as I never loved anyone in the way that I loved her. This love was new to me. I love her to this day.

I was still living with Jenny, who became Aunt Jenny. As our third lease together was coming to an end, Sean asked me to move in. We had a garage sale, and I sold most of my furniture knowing his home (our home) was fully furnished. Eva and I only got closer. We had her 5 days a week, so I was considered her stepmom. I picked her up and dropped her off at daycare, fed her and bathed her. Sean never asked me to do any of those things. I volunteered, as I loved being a family. Over the next year and a half, Eva was speaking full sentences and we had potty trained her. My mother had become Grandma Trudi and my sister was Aunt Colleen.

I'll never forget the night Eva and I were brushing our teeth and she noticed the scar on my chest. Of course, the scar on my chest was from my multiple heart surgeries. She said, "What's that Kafween?" I told her it was a scar. I don't remember my exact explanation, but I know I didn't share it was from surgery, as she was only 3 and a half and I didn't want to scare her. I asked her if it was ugly. I will never forget her response. She replied immediately, "No it's beautiful." That, for sure, lives in my heart to this day. I always knew she was a special little girl.

Sean was a good man, but every couple has ups and downs. Ours was no different, and, eventually, led us to couples therapy as we tried to work things out. I am sure my anxiety and depression affected our relationship. I was not happy with my job at Dreams, and I am sure Sean brought some obstacles to the table as well. He and I are good people and we never cheated. It just didn't work out. I had pushed him away with past issues I had not worked on. That was my part. He had his. We grew apart but there is mutual compassion for each other, and we will always remain cordial. He is married today and if there is a "one that got away," he was the one I let go.

We ended things in April just as Eva was turning 4 years old in 2014. We had our biggest fight ever and couldn't recover from it. It was too much, and it was too late. I remember we sat outside our apartment one night crying. He told me, "Kathleen, you had me. I was all yours and you lost me." He didn't say it to be hurtful. He was so sad; we both were sad and crying. I had successfully pushed him away like I had done before in some past relationships.

Although it had been coming, it was still devastating. I was losing my family and I was losing the only daughter I have ever known. I was losing Sean. I was losing my two best friends. Sean was kind and he told me there was no rush to move out, but I didn't stay too long. I found a place closer to Dreams. I think he helped me move. I took all my stuff, except for a decanter and set of four wine glasses that he swore was his. (It was mine but I wasn't going to fight.) I took my broken heart and it ached physically. I ached emotionally. To this day, I believe heart surgery (and I have had more than one) has a quicker recovery time then a broken heart from a break up when you love somebody. I loved Sean, and I am so thankful for our time together.

Journal Prompt

"Trust happiness, sometimes it's hard to trust happiness when you know it can be taken away in a second." - Unknown

Write about a time in your life when you were at your happiest. How did this bring you Zen?

_____

_____

_____

_____

_____

"It's hard to turn the page when you know someone won't be in the next chapter, but the story must go on."

–Thomas Wilder

When I left Sean, I moved in with two Columbian ladies who both worked for Dreams as well. The condo was beautiful, the amenities were great, and I used the pool, the clubhouse, and the gym often. We had armed security, which made me feel safe, and I made friends with a couple of them. I missed Sean and Eva dearly. I remember how quiet the condo felt. I had gone from a loving family home to living with strangers. The ladies and I had opposite schedules, so there was a lot of quiet time at the condo. I tried to keep busy.

I learned some more Spanish when I was living there. One of my roommates only spoke Spanish so we would communicate through my broken Spanish. My other roommate spoke English and was much friendlier and we would go for walks together.

I was still only part-time at Dreams. It was, and is to this day, hard to get a full-time position as a server, at least in the better restaurants. I was no longer at the Famous Cheesecake. I left when Sean and I moved in together. That was his career. He had been with the company for years and although we had no issue working with each other, I felt it was best that I let him work at the restaurant alone.

When I was living with Sean, I was able to work at Dreams without a second job. Since I had moved out, it was time for me to get a second job again. I went back to 'Caribbean Soft Wind, but at a different location. This store was not as busy, but I was back with the company and I knew that I wanted to work at the company's other restaurant, Summer Nights.

Except for missing Sean and Eva, it was nice living with the Columbian ladies. I loved the space I had. It was private and comfortable, and I had an entire side of the condo. I had a large master bedroom with 2 large closets that formed a small hallway leading to a private his-and-hers bathroom. The price was good, too.

My friend Jenny came over often with our friend Dr. G. Jenny and I had met Dr. G a couple years before while playing trivia at a local bar. Dr. G was a character. He was an older man approaching his 70s. Everyone knew and loved Dr. G. We all called him that because he had been a professor with a PhD at a well-known Florida college. He was always telling jokes and making people laugh. Dr. G was smart and witty. He liked his drinks and the crowds, and the bartenders all loved him and called him by name.

When Sean and I first broke up, I was really sad. I didn't go out much, but Dr. G helped me get my Zen back. He was like a mentor, father, and friend all in one. He told me I had to get out of the house and start having fun again, so he brought me on to his live trivia team. When Jenny and I had first met him, we were playing a video-like trivia game at our favorite local bar. We all had our own trivia TV controllers and we played on a screen against each other with friends and strangers.

Live trivia was something totally different, as it has a DJ host that reads out questions on a microphone and keeps score. Groups of people gather and form teams. Most teams play weekly and have fun group names. We had a name, and everyone knew it because it was often that we placed in 1st, 2nd and 3rd, winning prizes. Our team included people of all ages, including 3 PhDs, one of whom was Dr. G. We had people participating from every theme park in Orlando. There were college kids on our team as well as plenty of people over 50. Everyone was included on our team, and it was a normal event to bring a friend or have a neighbor stop by to play. We even became friends with the teams we played against. It was a friendly competition and was always a super positive way to have fun and meet people.

Dr. G and Jenny would come over to the condo and we would play pool in the clubhouse or lay out by the swimming pool and tan. Some days, we would watch TV in the clubhouse and work out in the gym - whatever we did, we always had a good time.

"If it doesn't nourish your soul, get rid of it."
-Sarah Bolen

Eventually, the Columbian ladies were ready for a move, but I was not going with them. I had met a girl at Caribbean Soft Wind who was looking for a roommate. She had a 3-bedroom apartment, and it was very close to the restaurant. There were 4 of us in that 3-bedroom apartment. She and her boyfriend shared a room then another girl and I each had our own rooms and shared a bathroom. It seemed like it would work.

It was pretty quick that I determined this wasn't the place for me. I woke up one morning to discover a strange young man sleeping on the couch in the living room. This became a regular occurrence. I put a lock on my door. My male roommate would go out every night drinking. There was some pill popping and pot smoking as well. I have no issue with anyone smoking pot. Just saying, at the time, it was illegal. I was not happy and did not feel safe and I told my friends what was going on.

The last straw was learning that my male roommate was using our rent money for his parties. We apparently were going to be evicted. Thank goodness I was just renting a room and not on the lease. I asked him to give me my money back and luckily, I got my first month's rent back because he had not cashed the check. The rest of the money was probably up his nose or down his throat. Regardless of the way he used our money, the best thing was that I got out before anything else happened.

Dr. G was kind enough to offer me a temporary room in his 4-bedroom house in Dr. Phillips, Florida, a very nice part of Orlando. He lived alone. It was in a good area and close to everything. The restaurant I wanted to transfer to, Summer Nights, was just 5 minutes away from the house, and it was still a quick commute to Dreams. I felt very safe with Dr. G. This was perfect. This was Zen.

It is important that you feel comfortable in your home, as it should be a place where you can constantly find Zen. It is important. "If it doesn't nourish your soul, get rid of it." Place items around your home that make you smile. Pictures of loved ones, knick knacks and candles can bring a sense of happy Zen. Clear your clutter! I know you have heard this one before, but it is true. Get rid of the old that is no longer of use so that you can invite the new. Whenever I have moved, I have taken it as an opportunity to de-clutter. We acquire so much stuff over the years that we just don't need.

Playing soothing music, whether it is rap or Enya, evokes a Zen mood as well. If your house is loud, take a candle and a glass of wine into the bathroom and take a bubble bath. Close the door to the noise and drift into a calm space. Let yourself have a little Zen every day. If 5 minutes is all you have, then take those 5 minutes and enjoy them. Have a little chocolate or ice cream. Do something for yourself.

Meditation

"Give yourself a dose of love, and then listen with compassion to what your heart tells you." ------Susan Bernstein

In this meditation, I really want you to relax and let your guides speak to you. Get into a comfortable position. Close your eyes. I want you to breathe in deep and let out a sigh, 3 times.

Then take at least 2 deep breaths while counting. Breathe in for the count of 10, hold for a count of 2 and exhale for the count of 8. Now let your breathing slow on its own. Let thoughts come and go. Picture a gold light around you, harnessing positive energy. Let your mind drift to self-care and self-love. What are you being guided toward?

"In a world of algorithms, hashtags and followers, know the true importance of human connection"

-Unknown

Dr. G had never had a roommate. He didn't need one and he never really wanted one. He was very happy with his lifestyle. He played tennis three times a week, did happy hour five times a week, and played live trivia at least once a week. Dr. G also had girlfriends. Yes, multiple. He would date often. All the women were in his age group. Dr. G had annual passes to every theme park in Orlando. He attended the food and wine festivals, concerts, art exhibits, flower and garden festivals, and holiday events

His schedule was full, and this was just when he was in Orlando. He spent plenty of time traveling to see family all over the United States. He had a small home and a boat in South Florida where he did a lot of fishing. He also fished in Alaska at least once a year and the fish he caught in Alaska he would mail home to Orlando.

Dr. G was financially comfortable, but he was very modest with his money. He never spent much. His home was humble, as were his car and his clothes. He preferred happy hour prices to regular prices and would work his schedule around those. He even took his dates to happy hour. Happy hour food was his dinner when he wasn't eating at home.

We got along very well, and he called our relationship symbiotic. Even though our age difference was quite large, we were like best friends. He became my personal mentor and remains a best friend and father figure. We would play trivia, go out to dinner with friends, go to the theme parks, etc. Our friends knew us, and they had known that we had been friends for years. Those that didn't know us well whispered about me being a gold digger.' At times, this was hurtful, but it was more funny than anything and we joked about it a lot. He was never inappropriate with me and our intentions for each other were of honest friendship. I looked out for him and he looked out for me.

Living with a retired college professor was great because I was able to learn things from a very brilliant man. Dr. G had a lot of wise advice that he shared with people he cared about. One of his beliefs was that life was fair. He would say, "You get what you get to learn a lesson."

I moved in, in October. My birthday is November 1. Then, of course, Christmas is in December. So, Dr. G said I should stay for a few months. The plan was I would move out in January.

I got my transfer to Summer Nights. It was great. Again, this corporate company was great to work for and I met some great people working there. I enjoy serving and it is addictive. Not only is there cash in your pocket but it is fast moving. I feel like, for me, it brought me Zen in regard to my anxiety and depression. When you are in a restaurant serving people you really must be fully present. You're taking orders for one table while delivering desserts at another. You don't have time to think about personal problems.

Dr. G and I celebrated my birthday and the holidays, and, in January, I found a place to live. I was going to move in with my friend Joe who lived right outside Orlando. This would make my commute longer, so Jenny and Dr. G had a talk. They said this move was not the right decision. Dr. G then told me, "I don't mind having you here."

I responded, "I don't mind being here."

From that moment on, we became full-time roommates.

The experience of living with Dr. G is hard to put into words. I was so blessed that we had that time together. I will always love him, as he was an important part of my life. Through living with him, I was able to learn so much about life. He had so much experience, wisdom, and joy to share. We laughed together all the time. His motto was, "Life is too short to be unhappy or stressed." He believed that we get what we give. Dr. G taught me about forgiveness and love. Love for family and yourself. We would tell each other "I love you" every day. Johnny Cash was his favorite singer and he loved social media.

One of my favorite memories is the day he had surgery on his wrist. It was an outpatient procedure, but he was put on strong medication, so I had to sign him out, taking responsibility for him for 24 hours. He and I were instructed that he was not able to make financial decisions, sign important paperwork, etc. I took him home and made sure he was comfortable. He was in his recliner in the living room and had the TV on as well as his laptop and iPad. I told him I was going to take a nap. Right before I laid down, I decided to check my social media just to see what was going on in the world. I noticed that Dr. G had a new post. In the post, he declared that he was home and resting after his surgery. Not only did he check in, but he listed our full home address on his public page! I went running into the living room. I knew the meds were working. He was able to delete our address before we had any stalkers come by.

While I lived with Dr. G, I was happy. I enjoyed my jobs at Dreams and Summer Nights. The house was definitely Zen. He allowed me to decorate for every season and in between. I would have fresh flowers on the kitchen table and candles. I used bright colors in the summer and autumn colors in the fall. During the holidays, I would really decorate, as we loved to celebrate birthdays and holidays.

I was able to practice several of my Zen techniques, like yoga. There was an extra living room that I made my yoga studio. I would play workout videos. I even got Dr. G into yoga. We would do yoga in the house, and we would also attend classes at the local gym.

I would light candles, put music on and I was able to decorate my personal room in colors I enjoyed. I read books, painted, watched TV, and traveled to New Jersey and New York to see my family. Even on hard days at work, Zen was pretty easy to find with Dr .G. He would let me vent to him. At the time, I was also in therapy, so I was working hard with my therapist on past and present healing. When you have depression and anxiety, it is a full-time job on its own. Seeking and achieving Zen can save your life when things get dark.

I was single when I lived with Dr. G but not too lonely. I was living with my best friend, and we always had a great time together. There were times that I worried about how close we were because of our age but our age difference did not bother me. What did bother me, at times, was thinking about losing him to old age. I came to rely on him. We were platonic companions. We had no secrets, and nothing was off topic. I could tell him anything. He could tell me anything. We really shared so much. He had known all about Sean and was now helping me get back into the dating world.

As I said, Dr. G had a very active dating life with women of his own age. He was on several dating sites and it was not unusual for him to have a happy hour dinner date one night and a lunch date the next day. I remember one night, when I first moved in, he walked past my bedroom door with a backpack on, pacing back and forth. Finally, he looked at me and said, "I'm going on a sleepover." He was such a character. The ladies loved him.

Things changed a little in 2016, as that was the year he met Marie. I believe to this day that Marie was the love of his life. When they first started dating, Marie did not know that Dr. G had a roommate. Upon finding out, she was a little curious about the woman living in his house. Just as others in the past assumed there might be something romantic going on with us, I think that thought may have crossed her mind as well. One day, he asked me to go to a concert at an aquarium theme park with him, where he was meeting Marie. I knew she was different immediately when he asked me to meet her because he really didn't care what people thought about us. It was important to him that I meet Marie so she would feel more comfortable.

I remember seeing Marie for the first time. She was/is a stunning woman. Marie's elegance goes far beyond her physical beauty. Her grace and style are part of her soul. She was a delight, so warm and friendly, and we genuinely enjoyed getting to know each other. I could see why Dr. G liked her so much. In fact, he was smitten. From that time on, the only sleepovers he had were with Marie. They enjoyed each other's company so much. It was such a beautiful love story to watch.

Dr. G passed away in 2019. He will always be in my heart, and I will always love him.

Journal Prompt

"As hard as it is to feel pain, it is much harder to feel nothing."
-Harold Cooper (The Blacklist)

What is a former relationship that you still cherish to this day?
What fond memories of this person bring you Zen?

_____

_____

_____

_____

_____

"Last night I practiced self-care by eating cinnamon toast crunch in bed and letting the sugar crumbs in my sheets exfoliate my legs."

-Isabel Steckel.

While I was working at World Dreams, I had the opportunity to move in with a friend closer to the parks and resorts and save money on my commute. It had been almost three years and it was time to move out of Dr. G's house. It was actually very painful, as I loved him so much that it was like leaving a parent's nest. I had been so happy and safe there. It was time to spread my wings and Dr. G agreed. That did not stop us from crying. It was such a sad transition for us as we said goodbye to a special chapter in both our lives.

I moved in with my friend Kelly. It was January 2017, a new year with brand new opportunities. This was going to be my year; I was excited. I moved closer to Dreams and had some money in the bank. The biggest excitement I had was signing my book contract with Sean at That Guy's House.

> *"Sometimes the only way to catch your breath is to lose it completely."*
>
> –Tyler Knott Gregson

After 4 years of being single, I was ready to allow another person into my life when I met Keith in December of 2016. We had a lot of mutual acquaintances, so I knew a little bit about him. We both worked at Dreams. We never worked together, as we worked at two separate restaurants. I worked with the mother of his child, so I knew when she was in a new relationship and Keith was single. She and I were not friends; we were simply coworkers. So, I don't consider myself as breaking girl code in this situation. However, starting a relationship like this was not a Zen-like move. I should have known that peace would be hard to achieve with other parties involved.

It would be a disservice to myself and you if I did not include him in this book. I did debate whether to or not. He was a big lesson, a hard lesson and certainly not my favorite lesson.

I will try as hard as possible not to speak ill of him because he is human, and I still keep the good parts of him tucked somewhere in my heart. Hurt people, hurt people and this fragile human has been hurting his whole life. I wish him healing, love and Zen. This is a piece of our story. I invite you in.

Is love a distraction? For me it can be. Love also brings us Zen. Real love, true love brings comfort and peace. With that also comes vulnerability, lessons, and healing. I am someone who puts others first, which can be a downfall. Sometimes I put the wrong ones on a pedestal.

Through meditation recently I was told that it is time to stop putting people on pedestals. I must love Kathleen, as loving yourself brings Zen. You must love yourself. This is so important and essential to living a healthy, well-balanced life. "Talk to yourself like you would talk to someone you love." -Unknown

Every so often I would play on a hospitality bowling league with my friend Clint. Keith was on another bowling team and we never crossed paths at the bowling alley until a night in late December of 2016. My friend Ryan was a substitute on Keith's team that night and when he walked in, I was a couple Moscow mules deep. I knew who he was and asked Ryan if he was single. He said he was. I approached Keith and he bought me a drink. We chatted and flirted the whole night, and I could feel a connection right away. We had things in common besides finding each other attractive. I gave Keith my phone number. It was only a few days from Christmas.

Keith texted me January 2 and asked me out, but I almost didn't go on the date, as I didn't know if I was really looking for anything. He took me to one of my favorite restaurants, located on International Drive in Orlando. It's a trendy restaurant and very popular with the tourists and the locals.

Keith and I spoke openly, and I was very comfortable around him. He was a single father, which I had already known. We both worked at Dreams and knew a lot of the same people. Our conversation was surprising, and I certainly did not expect it. The amount we had in common would have been overwhelming if it didn't feel like fate. It was really something I had not experienced with anyone, not on this level, not this extreme.

Keith and I both had alcoholic fathers but not just the kind who remain home and create an uncomfortable living situation. We had alcoholic fathers who had to leave our homes and us to get professional help. Keith's father had gone to prison for his drunken mistakes and my dad went to rehab for what seemed to be my entire junior year of high school. It was only about 6 months, but in my mind it seemed forever. Today, my dad is over 25 years sober, and I could not be prouder to call my dad my best friend. Keith's father also got his life together and is a good guy. They do not have a relationship today but every so often they speak and try.

Keith and I also have very strong mothers who were our strength, as we both grew up with birth defects that required extensive surgeries. For me, I was born with a congenital heart defect that, over the years, required four heart surgeries. My first heart surgery was when I was 5 months old - it was an open-heart surgery. I would have 3 more heart surgeries, my last one when I was 18 years old. Keith and I both experienced an awkward adolescence, and we developed our self-esteem later in life. Keith and I both hid our physical defects from our classmates and friends. We hid our scars and both participated in sports. We actually had a pretty normal childhood, which is what our mothers both pushed for.

Keith and I also hid our family struggles. We did not share information about our fathers even with our closest friends when we were growing up. If I had a friend over at my house asking where my dad was, I simply explained his absence was due to a business trip. Absent fathers mold children differently, especially when they leave for a reason that could be viewed as shameful. Back in our day, getting help for alcohol and drug use was not viewed as it is today. Today, it is not only more acceptable to come out and admit you have a problem, but you are also usually quick to find support around you.

I was vulnerable with Keith and it was his vulnerability that had me deeply attracted to him. For a man with such a history, he seemed to be handling life very well. He had shared custody of his son. So, he had an 11-month-old baby on his own at least 3 days a week. His apartment was spotless. No dirty dishes, no overflowing laundry, and the bathroom was clean. He was a great cook and he loved to grill out by the pool. We had fun. We played board games together, listened to 80s music, went bowling and, of course, went to World Dreams with our free admission. The emotions he brought out of me was something I hadn't experienced in a long time. Keith was handsome, talented, and loving towards me. His work reputation was that of a composed, measured professional. He seemed like a real catch, but sometimes people are not what they seem.

Keith and I became equally smitten with each other. He asked me to move in the first two weeks of dating, but I think I waited two months, as I had just moved in with Kelly. Keith really needed a roommate to help pay bills and be more hands-on deck to take care of his son. I was unaware or ignoring that fact at the time. We rushed. I rushed. The train had left the station and I didn't know what I was in store for. Kelly did not support my decision. She was one of the first people to see through his manipulation, so she tried to get me to stay with her. Kelly knew exactly why he was rushing for me to move in. I was in a month-to-month lease with her and regrettably did not take her advice. It damaged our friendship. I was becoming blind to my reality.

Moving in was not a good idea, but I was highly distracted by our love or lust or fantasy.

Keith needed more help than I could give. He needed money so mine depleted. He had a son, so I became his main source of childcare for a 13-month-old baby. He needed a scapegoat when his world was falling apart. Someone to gaslight and yell at. Someone to project his pain onto. It was emotional abuse and was the worst relationship of my life, and I never saw it coming. We were two damaged human beings too damaged to help each other.

Keith took no interest in providing support for my anxiety and depression. In fact, he added to it. He saw my anxiety and depression as weakness. Being with him was one of the most painful times of my life. I always held on to hope that he would change back into the man he was in the beginning, the man I fell in love with. I would continue to support him emotionally and financially. I was confused and often left alone with my thoughts.

I would eventually discover that the man I fell in love with was an illusion and I was more in love with his potential than who he really was. The circle of arguments was an unhealthy addiction to us both. Our imperfections should have been our strengths. We would fight and make up over and over. I let him get away with things like belittling me. The only one who set the standard for how he could treat me was me, so, in a way, I allowed this. I wanted to keep him happy, so I bent over backwards. I thought he loved me, and I compromised the way I valued myself. I didn't challenge him often; I didn't want to lose him. It was just better to keep the peace.

We both claimed we were in love and he was promising to be better, to be nicer, and to drink less. He apologized over and over for his behavior.

I believed deep inside that he could change. I remembered the man he used to be. He was not difficult to get along with when I met him. He was charming and he had loved me. There was something real that had made me fall in love with him so quick and so strong. Our love was a dangerous love though, and even with the warning signs his love tempted me. This man had made me laugh and kissed me soft. There was a time when I really trusted him. I had to believe he was the man that I had introduced myself to in the bowling alley.

My dear friend Steve Sapiro said it to me best: "When you are in an unhealthy relationship, it is hard to be healthy yourself." When you sacrifice yourself for someone else, you sacrifice your Zen, your power, and your strength. That is exactly what I did, and I didn't realize it until it was too late. Our relationship bordered on abuse. It was mostly emotional abuse. I was blind to his control and I really wanted a happy ending.

During the time when I chose to stay with him and was too weak to leave him, I found Zen in several ways just to keep going. I found Zen in my candles (you know I love them) music, TV shows, books, our pool, and the gym. I would clean the house and do the laundry. I would take walks. I would spend time on the phone with friends but did not spend a lot of time with friends without Keith. I would do my yoga on my purple yoga mat in stretchy yoga pants. Yoga has truly been a life saver. Unfortunately, I found my Zen in drinking as well.

I was a pretty heavy drinker at that time and Keith was a really big drinker. Keith is probably an alcoholic, but I didn't see it at the time. He always had a 24-pack of beer in the house and the time of day he drank didn't matter. I started to follow suit at least from the afternoon on. Keith would have beer for breakfast at times and I accepted it. When I drank, I was more relaxed. We both were and we would get drunk together a lot. I hated drinking and I loved it at the same time, but I became pretty dependent on it.

Like I mentioned, I did find Zen in positive activities, too. I indulged in the simple things that brought me comfort. I have always been a big reader, so I was usually reading a book or two. Never doubt the power of temporary escape from a good book. I also watched a lot of TV. Some shows we even watched together and some good movies. He was into sci-fi; I am not but I did enjoy some of what he introduced me to. I found Zen working out and going to the pool. We found calm together grilling out at the apartment complex's BBQ. We found Zen in making love. It was addictive. Most of the time, it was really beautiful.

It wasn't always bad, which is another reason I put up with a lot. There were times he made me feel really good. I would convince myself that this was our real life - the good. The bad was just temporary. I wished he was the man he made himself out to be. Like I said, no relationship is perfect. We had our ups and downs, but I was initially in denial that we had more downs than anything. Keith had used me and lied to me, making me believe that he regretted his actions. He made me believe that things could work out for us.

I was around to teach his son to walk and that was one of our biggest joys. His son was adorable and had a great personality. Keith has partial custody and spent way too much time at court trying to fight for more custody, claiming his ex was an unfit mother. It was a strenuous time, and I was way too involved. He had roped me into a battle that wasn't mine and the stress this caused was tremendous. It really took a toll on my anxiety and depression, which he wanted nothing to do with. He left me on my own for that.

My meds and my therapy were something Keith really didn't want to be a part of. I wish that had been different. I felt like him participating in my therapy would be good for both of us as I wanted him to understand me, and I wanted to understand him.

What was really abusive was when he used my anxiety and depression against me. I remember during one of our volatile fights he took my medication out to the balcony and poured the pills loose in his hands. He emptied the bottle and threatened to throw it over the balcony, which would scatter all over the ground and be lost in the bushes. He had power over me once again. All I could see was the look of anger on his face as he looked directly into my eyes with his gorgeous blues that had suddenly turned dark grey. His expression looked evil. It was like he hated me. I felt I disgusted by him. Maybe it was me that brought out the worst in him? Was there something wrong with me that provoked him to act like this? So spiteful, so irrational.

This was an extreme behavior that I had never witnessed in him or anyone close to me until that night. I believed, at that moment, he could physically hurt me and, in the future, he would. I should have trusted my instincts. Learn from my mistakes and please trust yours. I felt my pulse quicken and, in that moment, I just wanted to jump out of my skin.

I didn't know how to react but, I believe he got the exact reaction he was looking for. I was left crying and begging him to stop. I was so scared. If I didn't have my medication, there would be complications. He was so incredibly cruel. I wouldn't have put it past him to carelessly and viciously dispose of my medication.

At the time maybe it was just a stunt or maybe I had told him what he wanted to hear. He handed my pills back to me and I felt relieved and foolish at the same time. I had put myself into this situation with Keith and did not see a way out. Either way, my medication was saved, but I knew he didn't love me. The sinking feeling physically hurt my stomach with this realization. As I took it all in, my head began to hurt. He cracked open a new beer and handed it to me, then he cracked open a fresh one of his own. I knew I had made a big mistake.

Even on my good days, memories from that night and other arguments we had would haunt me.

Sometimes it would take me a xanny (which I was prescribed) or two with a hot shower and a cold beer to calm my anxiety. Mixing drugs and alcohol was a dangerous way to self medicate.

I sobbed in the shower too many times to count. Concealer was my friend when the red around my eyes from crying lasted too long. I wore my makeup and smiled as a mask to all those around me. Many believed I was very happy.

One of the worst parts of our relationship was that I put all his priorities above mine. My writing suffered as I pushed it to the side to care for his son and nurse his drunken self-pity. Keith always felt that the world owed him more. He said he was afraid to succeed but lacked motivation. I began to see him as ugly (on the inside) snarky and sneaky.

Again, I was attracted to his potential. I stayed with him for many reasons. No one is perfect, and I believed in him and I was weak. He had a tough life and I made excuses for him. His story from his childhood, and the scars he carried, were so sad. He was a broken man and, of course, I thought I could heal him. I thought I could help him smile again and he would fall back in love with me and treat me well again. No relationship is perfect and just because we had problems didn't mean we couldn't fix them.

Keith was human, after all, and so was I. I have been awful to people before, so I knew what it was like to take your emotions out on people that didn't deserve it. A big difference from Keith and I was that I always had remorse for the people I hurt. He did not. I did not know the word for him at the time because I had never dated one, but he was and is a narcissist.

I was his scapegoat and in my mind it would get better. If only ... when "this" happens ... we will be happy again. Keith will be himself again and I would be able to return to myself and he would be the man I had fallen in love with at the beginning. The mystery man I had met at the end of 2016, who I allowed to enter my life at the beginning of 2017, had disappeared into a sad, angry man in the short few months after we began our journey together.

In January 2017, when we began dating, I had just signed my book contract and had money in the bank, a great job, and a new place to live. I was so excited that I had met this wonderful/wonderfully broken man. Little did I know it wouldn't be long until I lost everything - the most precious being my confidence, my self-esteem, my happiness, my Zen, and MYSELF.

My family and friends could see everything I couldn't. They could see how he was emotionally abusing and using me. They noticed how I changed, how my self-esteem had diminished and how my priorities had been pushed to the back burner. I had lost my joy and motivation, and I was not getting my Zen on. There were more bad days then good.

While stuck and blind for a long time in the darkness of this toxic relationship I must credit my family and friends for fighting for me to come back. I can't count how many times they all would say, "We want to see Kathleen again." I was not myself. I was lost. That girl was gone. If it were not for the support of my family and friends, I would not have survived, literally.

My friends and family were so worried they had an intervention with me. My brother and sister

came down to Florida from New Jersey and physically moved me out of his place. My parents provided rent for my new place. Without my family and friends to pull me out, figuratively and physically, I would not be where I am today, and I am forever grateful. My loved ones helped me get my Zen back. Never underestimate the Zen that loved ones will bring. When you feel like hiding the most, remember there are people you can rely on. It is never shameful to ask for help or to accept help. Sometimes that is exactly what we need.

Journal Prompt

"I keep going to the river when I pray." - Ella Henderson

What would you tell yourself about a past heartbreak? What do you know to be true that you didn't know a year ago? How does healing your past bring you Zen?

_____

_____

_____

_____

_____

"Do Something Today That Your Future Self Will Thank You For."

-Sean Patrick Flanery

So, you see, the past couple of years have added some new stories, some new trials and some new bursts of resilience. I could not survive without God, angels, the universe, and my friends and family. I reference my lessons to being on a rollercoaster because I find that to be very accurate.

The excitement, the fear, the nausea, the crying, the screaming, the laughter, the lows and highs, the twists and turns - that is a rollercoaster. Those are also the lessons in my life. Many seasons of my life. Sometimes I feel like I am going upside down and around, and other times I feel stuck like the ride attendant forgot about me.

Getting your Zen on can be as simple as having a cup of tea, lighting some incense or going shopping. It can be bigger, like getting on a plane and traveling to see someone special or backpacking overseas by yourself to experience the wonders of the world. It can be getting in the car to escape to the beach. It can be sitting in the grass in your backyard feeling the sun and the breeze.

Getting your Zen on should be a daily goal. It can last 2 minutes, 2 days or 200 days in a row. Please share with me the secret to 200 days of straight Zen if you find it! I need that too! Getting your Zen on is what you make it. It is your Zen that is completely unique to you. What you find that brings you joy and peace may be totally different then what I find are my own ideas of joy and peace. Again, I will take your advice if you can get your Zen on for 200 days straight!

Create your own magic! Not all of us can afford nice trips or the bottle of expensive champagne. Thank goodness for places like trendy health food stores with a very affordable wine and beer selection as well as snacks that are both healthy and tasty. By the way, I try not to drink to excess anymore, as I made that lifestyle change in 2019. I drank a lot when I was with Keith then I continued drinking heavy to heal from the aftermath. Today, I am happy to say that I no longer use alcohol to self medicate.

When I say to have a glass of wine and take a bath, I am not condoning to escape through a blackout or mask emotions to achieve your Zen. When I say to have a glass of wine, that is what I mean, a glass. Alright, you may have two.

Zen is available for everyone and for every budget. It actually costs nothing. For example, look at the sky, rainy or sunny, day or night. When the rain falls there is always a chance of a rainbow. When it rains, I am reminded that the earth is being cleansed; the grass, flowers and trees are being fed. When the storms come, they are powerful and exciting, even if frightening. They provide a different energy, and the lightning is a free show in the sky.

On sunny days, we can see things clearly and things are bright and happy. Colors are vibrant and we seem to have more energy. During a clear night when the stars are visible, we can stare up at the sky and the moon and imagine how big the universe is and how small our problems really are. So, go out in your own backyard or borrow a backyard from a friend. I am so blessed to this day that I have friends who let me borrow their pools, backyards and gyms for my Zen. I highly suggest you get your Zen on looking at the stars tonight. You are big but your problems are small. Remember, everything is temporary.

Journal Prompt

What are 5 of your go-to techniques you use to create happiness? To create your Zen?

They can include people, places and things, and, of course, pets.

_____

_____

_____

_____

_____

"I offer you my flaws and my service."
-Cyrus Bean (Scandal ABC)

I have tremendous support with my anxiety and depression because I speak about it. Vulnerability can be one of your strongest assets and one of your greatest bonding tools. Vulnerability brings us Zen because we invite people in. I believe most people have a desire to help one another. Sometimes we learn from others' mistakes. No one is perfect but we are all perfectly imperfect and as unique we are similar. They say not to compare yourself to others, but I think that is easier said than done, especially with social media today.

There is a fascination in success, and it is proven that the people you surround yourself with have a direct influence in your life. If you want to be successful then you must surround yourself with successful people. So, if you want light, love and Zen in your life, you must surround yourself with positive people who seek to achieve the same.

When we attract the right people in our lives, we can achieve a higher vibration. We can harness energy together to grow, learn, heal and find Zen. You may have experienced this through yoga or an athletic dance class. Maybe you have experienced this at church. When like-minded, positive people bond, that energy grows and lifts everyone involved. It is important to remember that we are not on this journey alone and that by using our resources, achieving Zen will become easier.

Your Zen is all about you and what you are looking to achieve in your calm and sacred space. Your Zen is personal, it is comfortable, it is tangible, it is real. However, you must create it and you must allow it. Resistance to good things can be in our nature. We must break down walls, be brave, be vulnerable and welcome acceptance.

Magnificent waterfalls and ocean waves delight my ears. We can find that in nature or even in music. Zen ignites all 5 of our senses. We can touch Zen when we pet the cat or dog. We can hear Zen through music. We can see Zen in the beauty of a child playing on the playground. We can taste Zen at an award-winning restaurant or in grandma's home cooking. We can smell Zen in a luscious garden, fresh apple pie coming out of a warm oven or scented candles. Yes, I love my scented candles.

I am on a budget so while I would love to do $40 candles and more all the time, I am just as happy with my $5 scented grocery store candles. I also love places like discounted goods for your home and clothing stores that let me find my Zen without draining my wallet. I can get my candles there (and a new purse).

Meditation

Find a moment to relax. Sit or lay down in a calm, quiet area. Set a time limit if you have to. Notice your body and your breath as you close your eyes. Let your thoughts come and go. Focus on your present breathing. Feel your stomach expand with every breath. Think about the things that bring you joy. Feel the Zen. Calm. Peaceful. Worries set aside. This is your time now, 5 minutes or 5 hours. A piece of peace, a piece of Zen. Inhale for count of 5, hold for count of 2, exhale for count of 5. Repeat as needed.

Did you have any thoughts during your meditation that you would like to share?

"Your life is your story, write well, edit often."
-Anonymous

I signed my publishing contract in January of 2017, and I expected to have my first book out that same year. The original title of this book was to be called "Enlighten up Honey," a phrase on my publisher's coffee mug. Throughout my life, many have seen me as an uplifter. I try to be an optimist. When people have issues, I like to help solve them or at least be there for them. I am guilty of hiding my own struggles but, in recent years, I have learned that vulnerability actually brings strength. It is ok to let the right people in. You certainly don't want to share everything with everyone. You need to find your tribe. These are like minded, compassionate and strong people you can trust. I encourage you to let some of your walls down and invite people in. Remember, being vulnerable requires strength. It also brings strength.

"Are we gladiators or are we bitches?"
-Scandal ABC

Honestly though, I am a Scorpio from northern New Jersey (25 minutes outside of NYC) and if it is warranted, some people say I am a bitch or have a temper. I'm emotional so being an imperfect uplifter is true. My spiritual truth, just like yours is love. I fight for the underdog and "respect the janitor the same as the CEO." I am above no job and no job is above me. My parents taught me that as business owners. They practiced what they preached, never asking an employee to do work that they wouldn't do themselves. I saw them do every job there was in the business, from driving trucks and answering phones like secretaries to cleaning the bathrooms. They were responsible for everything. They instilled in me never to ask someone to do something that you would not do yourself. I took this knowledge to Dreams, especially in the higher titles I held.

There was a time when I was impressed by titles. Of course, that was in my early 20s. I was engaged at 26 and my fiance was climbing the ranks at his company, so I decided to try the same at Dreams. I put in too many hours and it took a toll on our relationship. I was chasing what I thought was my dream, status and success. World Dreams LOVES to give titles! I don't think the compensation they offer for the titles they promote is fair. It is a lot lower than you would think.

When I got my first official title at Dreams, as facilitator of SIMS (safety in motion) classes, that was the beginning of it all. I taught Safety in Motion at both Dreams Nautical and Dreams Ocean resorts. Team members all over the resorts knew me and upper management was paying attention. I got a mentor and together we began to work on my professional plan. I was suddenly special and on the right path.

When I got my second official title of food and beverage coordinator, I was thrilled. This meant a transfer to a new location with a totally new role. It was exciting. I was going to Dream's Tropical water park. Once I was there, I oversaw the quick service locations, the mobile food carts and the bar. It was great. I was always moving. I had to visit each location, sometimes multiple times a day, to make sure things were running correctly. I was in charge of many tasks, such as giving breaks and bringing money for team members who needed change for their drawers or carts. During my training, I was put to work in each position I would be in charge of. If anyone needed a break or we were busy I could jump in and help at any time. I actually loved working the fryers in the back of the house at the quick service locations. I made really good French fries and chicken tenders. Burgers were fun, too.

The demand for performance at Dreams is high. As team members, we are numbers and replaceable because so many people want our jobs, so pay is minimal. I think my raise for my new position and amount of responsibility was a dollar or two above my associates. (Again, your sarcastic Jersey girl) I was so darn special.

There is even jealousy between our own departments. There was a woman who went for my job as a promotion, and she didn't get it. There were days when she really didn't like me for that reason. There are many times I have experienced the dog-eat-dog attitude. Yes, at Dreams, which I thought was, "The dreamiest place on our planet."

Today, I find the humblest people in high positions to be the most inspiring and worthy of respect. No one should ever forget where they came from or the blessings of special resources (aka parents, money, education, etc.) that placed them where they are today. We are all equal; however, not everyone has the same resources or understands the opportunity out there. It's funny how views change as we get older. What I thought was important then is something I don't want now. There was a time when I needed a title to feel worthy or successful.

I know I was also competing with my fiancé. Having a competition like that was not healthy for our relationship and it wasn't healthy for myself. It left little time for balance as I was always on the go. I found my Zen in my morning cafe mocha at the local coffee shop and my caffeine-free tea before bed. Few moments besides those were calm as I was always on the go go go!

As much as David and I encouraged each other to succeed, the long hours and dedication to our jobs left a small time for us and a lack of dedication to each other. I don't think my fiancé wanted me to work so hard. He wanted more time with me. He was prepared to be the breadwinner, but I was like a beast. I wanted to bring home the bacon just as bad. What a silly thing. So, I don't like titles for myself and, unless you are humble, I am not impressed by yours.

So back to "Enlighten Up Honey." I love this phrase and although it would have made a fine name for the book, I thought a phrase I personally use would be better! These are my personal stories that I am sharing with you after all, aren't they? Like I have previously mentioned, for years and years even before using the word Zen I have been asking people how they find daily peace in their lives. Then, of course, I would share some of my small remedies.

Sharing a remedy was like giving a prescription. I sent them home with something to complete that night. Some remedies were as simple as taking a bath, lighting a candle, taking deep breaths, or drinking a cup of tea. I am sure you have noticed these are some of my favorites. Some people required attention on the spot, and I have done deep breathing exercises with coworkers in elevators, kitchens and even in stairwells.

My first and always most important way to find peace is through prayer. I am not religious. As I have said, I don't like titles. I don't have a religion, but I have a very strong relationship with God and angels. I pray first thing in the morning and at night before bed. Throughout the day, I pray as well. God is #1 in my life.

It was actually a night that I was giving my mom a "Zen prescription" when the name of this book was born. "Get Your Zen On" was becoming my catch phrase and mantra. My mother and I were on the phone one night discussing her blood pressure. It was high. I told her, Mom pour yourself a glass of wine and get in the whirlpool ... and then ... just like that it came out again. "Mom, go get your Zen on." As soon as I hung up the phone, I repeated my signature mantra over and over out loud. "Get Your Zen On." The book's title was born, and I took the idea immediately to Sean. As my publisher, Sean has always been an inspiration and great support system. He is honest and caring. He loved the name, which in turn made me love it more.

I was eager to share some personal and unique experiences, like having 4 heart surgeries while having a completely active childhood. For example, I participated in gym class and exercised but I also was a cheerleader as well. I could have done other sports too, but I wasn't that coordinated.

It always took me more time on the cheer team to learn the routines, cheers and dances but that didn't stop me. I cheered in middle school and in college for a semester at Felician College in Lodi and Rutherford, New Jersey. I was home sick though. I ended up transferring to Ramapo College for my second semester and was a lot happier to be closer to home.

At Felician College, I was 45 minutes away from my family and I did not have a car. I was very homesick, so I chose to move home and attend Ramapo College in Mahwah, New Jersey, which was only 10 minutes away from our house. We all know how ironic this is now being that my family is in New Jersey and I moved to Florida in 2002/2003.

Upon signing my book contract, I knew it was time to be a true mental health advocate and speak openly about my anxiety and depression. Months before I signed, I got a semicolon tattoo on my wrist. Your life matters. Please look up projectsemicolon.com. I love my semicolon tattoo because it stands for hope and it is a symbol to people that they are not alone.

I was ready to share my parents' divorce and my failed engagement. I feel strongly that my parents' divorce had a deep impact on my relationships. I am sure it still does. As much healing and therapy I have had, I still have some to go. We all do, right? Your Jersey girl is perfectly imperfect, which I think many of you can relate to.

My move from New Jersey to Florida is and will be an exciting adventure for us to relive together. We will deeply explore that you can run anywhere but you cannot run away from yourself.

How naive I was in wanting to write a book about the power of the universe, not expecting the universe to respond. I literally thought I would use my past stories only. I had so much to share, so many experiences. I would just live my life and work and write from former experiences that I had. HAHA ... so shit hit the fan! That is the human way of saying the universe responded to my book deal and the title I picked for this book. The Universe said, "Kathleen SHOW US how YOU get YOUR ZEN on in daily situations today."

The Universe provided a larger story, bigger lessons, extraordinary new characters and mind-blowing plot twists. The last chapter suddenly became the first. I literally had a new life, and it was challenging. It was exciting for sure, terrifying often and simply devastating at times. As I signed my contract in January 2017, I never imagined that I was boarding life's rollercoaster for another crazy ride. Beauty and hope always remained.

Meditation

Let's dive deeper into this meditation. Once again, find a comfortable position. Close your eyes. Slow your breathing. Picture a protective gold light surrounding you. Work from your head to your toes, relaxing all the muscles in your body. There is no future, no past, just now. What do you feel? What do you see?

"Each difficult moment has the potential to open my eyes and my heart."

-Myla Kabat-Zinn

I have a large scar on my chest. My scar runs centered from just below my neck to about 2 inches above my belly button. There are some indents on my skin as well. They almost look like mini belly buttons or dimples. I have had 4 heart surgeries.

I was just a couple months old when my lungs filled with fluid, stopping me from breathing while my mom was giving me a bath. She shook me and got me to breathe again, and I was rushed to the hospital. I had been a healthy baby girl, born on November 1, 1979. No one knew at the time that I was born with a congenital heart defect.

My first of 4 heart surgeries was in 1980. I was only 5 months old and if I had been born a year earlier, I would not have had the chance to have this particular open-heart surgery and would not be here. Over the years, heart surgery and medicine in general has really evolved

For those of you in the medical field, or just curious I have, it is called Truncus Arteriosus Type A2. My mom can explain it like the back of her hand. I cannot. I ask her when I need it explained. Truncus Arteriosus is life threatening and, if untreated, most babies won't live more than a few months.

Truncus Arteriosus is very rare, like 1 out of every 33,000 births. Truncus Arteriosus accounts for 1 in 200 congenital heart defects. The cause of Truncus Arteriosus is unknown. This diagnosis changed our lives forever. My mother did not waste any time researching the best hospitals and best cardiologists in the United States. Columbia Presbyterian, known as New York-Presbyterian/Columbia, is still one of the top 5 hospitals in the nation today. That is where I had my heart surgeries. My mother had grown up in Suffern, New York, which was just outside NYC so she was familiar with the area. Located on 630 West 168th Street in New York, New York, my hospital was right in the middle of everything. The commute was difficult, as navigating around the city is not that easy to begin with. My mother made this commute like a pro. She brings positives to any situation and solutions to obstacles.

Growing up, I visited the hospital at least twice a year to have checkups. My checkups always consisted of an EKG (electrocardiogram). This non-invasive test can measure how fast the heart beats to how well the heart's chambers conduct electrical energy. An EKG is where electrodes (today they are sticker-like adhesives) are placed on your chest to record your heart's electrical signals. Your heart's electrical signals cause your heart to beat. In earlier years, the electrodes they used on your chest were like suction cups. They would pop off easily, making the procedure last quite long. However, it was important to get an accurate reading.

You are completely awake, and it is painless. Everyone's eyes, including mine, are glued to the computer monitor as it displays the signals as waves on the screen.

Another procedure that happened often was an echocardiogram (echo). This is very similar to a sonogram. During the echo, ultrasound from a handheld wand placed on your chest shows pictures of the heart's chambers and valves to evaluate the pumping action of the heart. This is also non-invasive but there is a lot of pressure placed on the chest, as the wand is pressed deep into the skin to get an accurate reading. Sometimes you have to lay flat; sometimes you roll over on your side. This is another test that can take some time because they want to get the right angles for the pictures they will show to the cardiologist. An average echo may last 40 minutes; mine is about an hour.

Another fun test for us cardiac patients is the stress test. This test is also called the exercise test or the treadmill test. That is what it is. Basically, they hook you up, put you on a treadmill and let you go until you can't anymore. This test monitors the patient's breathing, blood pressure and heart rhythm.

The last test that I would get often before a surgery is a cardiac catheterization. This is an invasive procedure used to diagnose and treat certain cardiovascular conditions. You are awake for this procedure. This test, for me, has been very painful. I hate it! During my "caths," a long, thin tube was inserted in the artery or vein in my groin. The tube traveled through blood vessels to my heart. With as much Novocain as they injected in my groin, I could still feel everything. As the heart is monitored on a big screen, a contrast dye is injected through the catheter to check for and monitor several things.

A cardiac catheterization is not considered a surgery because there is not a large incision and the recovery time is quick. The amount of information it provides the doctors is massive. The doctors are able to look for narrowed or blocked coronary arteries, check pressure in the four chambers of the heart, take oxygen content, evaluate the heart pumping, and look for defects in the valves or chambers of the heart.

When I was 16 years old, I had a cardiac cath that I will never forget. I think it was the most physical pain in my life. I was lying on the table in the middle of my cath and they were injecting the dye, which was always uncomfortable for me. When the dye is injected it feels gross and scary. I can't describe it. The dye heats my body up in certain places. For example, my throat feels like a hot liquid is sitting in it. So, while this normal uncomfortable situation is taking place, my doctor decides to do a procedure by using a balloon to open a valve or something. My mother was called in the waiting room. She gave the authorization for the procedure and next thing I knew there was a balloon in my heart expanding. I could feel everything, and it was excruciating. The procedure that was done that day pushed my heart surgery back a year or so.

I remember my last surgery most vividly. I had just turned 18, so I had to give consent myself. I was old enough and nervous enough to know I had to prepare myself physically and emotionally for the surgery. I made sure I ate well, slept and relaxed. I read books and spent time with my family.

"The Best is Still Unwritten"
- Natasha Beddingfield

When I was 18 years old and had my fourth heart surgery, my cardiologist told me that I would have to have heart surgery every 10 years. I remember that moment in her office; I said no in my head. It was more than not wanting to have surgery every 10 years. It just didn't make sense to me. With prayer and modern technology this would not be my life. This was not the life I was meant to live. I would not be sick forever. I had had enough.

When I was studying business at Ramapo College my beliefs were confirmed. I started to attract like-minded people and stumbled into Elaine's Feng Shui boutique in Ridgewood, The Purple Pear. Upon discovering many things, like Feng Shui, I learned that the mind/body connection was real. I always knew it was, but for the first time I was actually attracting these people and places into my life, and I was finding confirmation of such outside myself. It was amazing.

Alternative medicine in the United States was not very popular when I was growing up. If you were sick, you went to the doctor, not to an acupuncturist. Upon meeting my mentor Elaine, owner of the Purple Pear, I was introduced to energy healing like Reiki. I also read books about the mind/body connection. Many of the books I found on the shelves of the Purple Pear. This was my first real introduction to what I already knew to be true.

"The Patient's hopes are the physician's best ally."

- Norman Cousins

As humans, we need to be addressed on a physical and emotional level when it comes to our health. Our hearts do more than just pump blood and a true physician acknowledges this. We also have a spiritual, physiological and emotional heart. So, we need to be treated in a way that addresses us as a whole. Unfortunately, alternative medicine still has a discriminating stigma, but with the open-minded, the benefits speak for themselves.

Our bodies and our minds are connected. Ever notice that when you don't feel good emotionally, something physical usually follows and vice versa? My anxiety is often accompanied by stomach discomfort. With the mind/body connection, emotion, attitude and spirit affect our physical health.

"There is no false hope."

- Bernie Siegel

Now is the time that we must have the curiosity and courage to combine both worlds of Eastern and Western medicine. Scientific studies have shown that a healthy diet and lifestyle can influence the progression of illness. Sometimes a certain diet and healthy lifestyle can even reverse the effects of illness on the body. For this reason, patients like me have to be active in our own overall health. It is our responsibility to give ourselves all the ways possible for healing and why wouldn't we want to? Imagine avoiding a surgery by eating broccoli once a week. I said imagine! We might not be at that level but there are a lot of options that help prevent further ailments and deterioration of our bodies.

I like to explore alternative medicine methods as well as traditional medicine. I think the best idea is to blend them both. I want every opportunity available as possible for healing my body. Don't you want that for yours? Reality is that modern medicine does not solve or understand all of our human illness.

For years, doctors were taught to detach from their patients. Thankfully, this is more in the past. Today, we are not just a number or diagnosis. We patients have become human to our physicians.

In a hospital or doctor's office, it is so easy and completely normal to feel anxious, hopeless and depressed when facing a diagnosis. We need to be treated physically, of course, but we cannot forget to treat ourselves emotionally as well. The mind is a powerful thing. I know how easy it is to slip into depression.

Simple techniques, such as a breathing exercise, can help us battle illness as well as normal daily stress. Personally, I rely on breathing exercises often to calm my daily anxiety. My four heart surgeries and other life lessons propelled my journey to never underestimate the mind's role in healing the body. We need to do whatever is in our power to make ourselves healthy and whole.

I truly believe that it is the whole package, every technique from surgery and chemo to deep breathing and meditation. I want to use what works. It doesn't matter to me whether it is eastern or western medicine. It certainly doesn't matter to me if your opinion or belief is different. It wasn't that long ago that a study showed 7 out of 10 users of alternative medicine never even told their physician about their alternative treatments, techniques and consultations. This is almost silly that people are embarrassed or in fear of judgment for such practices. Isn't optimal health the ultimate goal for everyone? We should be working together as a team. If you want to use alternative medicine and your physician doesn't support this, you may want to consider another doctor.

When we visit our general care physician and need another doctor with a different set of skills, we are given a recommendation. Different studies and talents are recommended all the time for specific care. For example, if I were to get pregnant, I would have a team of doctors that would have to work together, combining their specialty skills to ensure a healthy pregnancy. Because of my heart history, I would need my cardiologist, gynecologist, and general care to be on the same page and communicate properly. I do not have any children and have never been pregnant, but I have always been a high risk and remain so if that time ever comes. Honestly, I have always wanted children, so I have had these discussions with my doctors before. Now, at my age, I have accepted that it may not be in the cards for me to have a child naturally. I have not given up on adoption though. Maybe even a surrogate? Any volunteers?

When healing our bodies, we cannot separate our emotional and spiritual life. I do not shun conventional medicine. For broken bones, deep cuts, etc. I would obviously go to the emergency room immediately. For common minor ailments like colds and headaches, I just try to heal myself with fluids like tea and herbs like Echinacea. It takes me hours with a headache to give in and reach for a pain reliever. Even though I take medication for anxiety and depression, I really don't like taking medication at all.

Here in the 21st century we are in the age of the quick fix. The average person believes that modern medicine can fix almost anything. People are still passive followers of their doctors. I want to reiterate that we need to be a team. We need to be active participants on our journey to health.

As a heart surgery patient, I have had a unique experience experimenting with such techniques. It is easy to pop a pill for a headache or really any ailment. We can no longer ignore that there are healthier things that might work too. There is certainly no harm in trying. I remember watching Oprah years ago learning that sometimes the glass of water we take with a pain reliever for a headache can be the cure. Sometimes a headache comes about because we are dehydrated. A simple glass of water can alleviate the pain.

There is overwhelming evidence that our immune systems are affected by our mind as well as our emotions. Depression, anxiety, divorce, a loss of a job and loneliness along with other stressful situations lowers our immunity. We all know that when our immunity is low that leaves us open for disease. Around the world, this is being studied in labs. Ongoing research is showing how our brains and bodies are connected. We have all heard the story of someone dying from a broken heart. If you need to, just watch "The Notebook." There are social aspects involved as well as chemical reasons behind our emotions. For me, I have experienced the childhood trauma of divorce. I have also been clinically dead four times. When you are placed on a heart and lung machine during heart surgery, that can certainly alter the chemicals in your brain.

Depression is strongly linked to heart surgery patients. Sometimes it's just the idea that our heart is not keeping up with us. It is a common thought or feeling that our bodies are giving up on us. This can be true in other emotions with other diseases.

Regular stresses, such as work, relationships and time of day, can influence our moods, therefore affecting our bodies. On the opposite end, such things as having healthy relationships with friends and family really play a big role in our positive mood and good health. Social intimacy is proven to relieve loneliness and depression.

Living with balance is not only important, it is essential. To have balance in this chaotic stressful beautiful world we must come up with ways to reduce stress in a healthy way. Instead of popping a pill for your latest ailment why not try a cup of herbal tea, yoga, or a massage? These may bring relief without a risk of side effects that are possible with all drugs.

When you are sick or diagnosed with a medical condition your first reaction may be panic. After the panic you need to plan. Implementing a lifestyle change may help reduce or heal the condition. Lifestyle changes are not always easy, but they literally can save your life.

Nutrition plays a major role in our mental and physical health. You have heard the saying, "You are what you eat." You may want to hire a nutritionist or dietician. You can also do your own research. My biggest advice is drink lots of water and stay away from sugar. That is my advice, but at this very moment in my own life I am not staying away from sugar. So be easy on yourself; it doesn't happen overnight. I can tell you that I drink plenty of water and I love herbal tea. I have an unhealthy addiction to ice cream!

Something that has helped me with my mental health, which I do believe connects to my physical health is therapy. Having a trusted therapist that can listen confidentially and can implement healing techniques from past emotional traumas is a great resource. I completely recommend it! Now, if you are not satisfied or do not vibe well with a therapist, don't be discouraged. It may take you a couple visits with different counselors to find the one you fit with. It is important that you feel comfortable and safe with a therapist.

Music is another wonderful resource. I am sure there is a genre for everyone. For many people, music is a release. Whether I am singing or dancing to my favorite music, I do feel an escape. Whether you play an instrument, sing and or dance it is certainly de-stressing to jam out.

Another relaxation technique that has worked for me is yoga and even more so Les Mill's Bodyflow. This is an exercise that blends yoga, Pilates and tai chi into a great workout for your mind, body and soul. Les Mills On Demand offers these Bodyflow workout videos. You can also find free yoga videos on YouTube. You don't even need a yoga mat. Use a towel or just work out on your carpet. Anything that gets the blood flowing and the body moving is going to be good for you. This boost in serotonin will bring you more happiness naturally.

Let's try something. Take three deep breaths. Inhale through your nose and breathe out your mouth. Stretch your arms all the way up, hands toward the ceiling. You should feel slightly more relaxed. What do you think?

Meditation

Get into your comfortable spot. Again, calm and quiet, and if you need to set an alarm do, so now. Let your body lead you. You are the #1 person in your life and don't forget it. This time is for you. Close your eyes. Listen to your breath. Focus on your stomach expanding with each breath. Be kind with your wandering mind. When you drift, just bring yourself back and focus. Remember this takes practice. What did you realize from this meditation?

My Mother, My Hero

I don't remember much about my early heart surgeries. My first heart surgery was when I was 5 months old and my last was when I was 18. During my third heart surgery, I have happy memories of getting ice cream from the nurses and my stepfather visiting me, bringing with him a ginormous stuffed animal. It was a black cat with long hair. Also, I found a snail in the garden and somehow made it my pet. I had pet rocks too. I had a great outlook and a great imagination, which I owe to my mother. I don't know how she did it, but she was always upbeat with me. She never let me see her fear, exhaustion, or sadness. She carried that on her own. I am thankful she was able to lean on my stepfather for support during my later surgeries.

When I was 18 things got real. I wasn't a child anymore and I knew exactly what was going on. I was having heart surgery, or I was going to die. For the first time, it was my decision to make and sign the appropriate documents giving consent. I remember asking what happens if I don't have the surgery. The doctors were honest.

My mother was always my rock. She had been through this many times before and she was guiding me along the way. I knew most of what to expect, a lot of needles, IVs and physical pain. I knew that to prepare for the surgery I had to be mentally and physically healthy. I spent time with friends and spent as much time being normal as possible. I tried not to stress out and stay positive. I knew I had to eat well. I was blessed, and we always had healthy meals at home, but that didn't keep me away from junk food, ice cream and pop tarts.

The night before my surgery my friend Ryan called and asked if there was anything he could bring me before I had to stop my food consumption for the surgery. He brought me some of my favorite ice cream. It was perfect. To this day, ice cream is still an emotional go to for me. I know it 100% helped that night!

THE HEART SURGERY

*"Any sufficiently advanced technology is
indistinguishable from magic."*

- Arthur C. Clarke

I would like to provide you with an authentic description of my last heart surgery. In doing so, this part of the story may be too graphic for some. If you need to skip ahead, that is totally understandable. I just want to give you fair warning.

One of the scariest things surrounding heart surgery is your lack of control. As patients, we give all the control to our trusted doctors in hopes that they will be able to fix us. This is why I am open to healing without a scalpel if possible. Even though we are dying, we risk immediate death with this surgery. I must tell you, though, the survival rate is very high and worrying doesn't help anyone.

Before surgery, you are injected with drugs, most to sedate you. Another example of learning how powerful the human mind is, is when I was being taken to the operating room and asked to use the bathroom. As they wheeled me down the hall, we stopped. Even with my body full of these pre-surgery drugs, I was able to get up and walk to the bathroom on my own. My mother and the nurses were amazed.

Upon entering the operating room, loved ones are left at the door. This is not an easy thing. You don't say "goodbye." Instead, you say, "I will see you when you wake up." As a patient, I was scared and felt alone, even with all the medical staff around me. As a parent, I can only imagine. My mother is one of the strongest people I know. She has been through this 4 times with me. My mom is all too familiar with the procedures, long waits, hospital food, nurses, doctors and orderlies. She has learned the professional medical terms because it was important to her. It is not easy to learn to speak and understand "Grey's Anatomy" like we pretend it is. She has endured so much. I am so blessed that she remains by my side.

It's a weird sensation being in an operating room - the bright lights, the machines, the IV in your arm and the conversation. Everyone is in blue gowns, gloved and masked. Medical staff are trying to keep you calm knowing you are scared. They speak to you. They spoke to me, explained how they would put me to sleep, and it would be quick and painless.

So, they did. They gave me a gas anesthetic to inhale; I tried to relax and not fight that I was being put under. I breathed in, and in just a few breaths, my body began to tingle. My sight started to blur with each breath as did the conversations around me. Before my surgeon, Dr. Quagbar, got started, I had been in a deep sleep for about 20 minutes.

When I was under, my surgeon felt with his hand for the center of my breastbone. My ribs would be spread open to expose my heart. With what they call a "ten blade," he began the incision right below my neck. Most surgeons have to cut along an imaginary line, but with my previous surgeries, it was easy for him to slice and slide the blade neatly down to just above my belly button. The skin splits apart like a zipper. In fact, heart surgery patients often refer to each other as being in the "zipper club."

Once the chest was sliced, it was ready for my ribs to be spread. At this point, the anesthesiologist "drops the lungs," which means they temporarily stop the breathing. My heart was connected to a heart and lung machine. This machine completely takes over the function of the heart and lungs.

Dr. Quagbar and his assistant pulled on the bone he had just divided, and my chest opened. From there, the scientific magic took place. My heart was temporarily stopped so that my surgeon could work on my still heart. Stopping the heart is a 30-to-90-minute process. The bright red blood rushed through tubes and my heart was left motionless.

I am forever grateful to my surgeon and the medical staff. The work they do is a miracle and I do believe is guided by God and angels. I believe in the power of prayer. A strong dose of prayer is the best and oldest healing therapy that I have used.

When you wake up you are surrounded by monitors. There are tubes and wires connected to your body. There are two to three tubes in the chest to drain fluid from the area around the heart. These are where the dimples on my chest come from. There are intravenous (IV) tubes supplying the body with fluids. There is also a catheter (thin tube) placed in the bladder to remove urine.

People asked how I was feeling but I had limited communication skills. I was attached to machines that were monitoring my heart. Nurses were nearby if I needed help. I was unable to speak right away because I was intubated, so I put on my game face. As scared as I was, I also tried to be brave for those around me. My family took turns attending to my needs, such as encouraging me to eat. I had no problem eating ice cream.

The surgery batters a patient's mind and body. That is why a lot of heart surgery patients have depression. Having heart surgery can leave you feeling physically and emotionally vulnerable. We know we have almost died. I have faced my own mortality. In fact, the morning of my surgery I played Queen's "Bohemian Rhapsody" and sang loudly, "I don't want to die, I sometimes wish I'd never been born at all."

The heart and lung machine can also affect the chemical balance of the brain. This can induce a biochemical depression. My depression is definitely a chemical imbalance. Whether or not it is from my surgeries, I don't know.

The heart is the center of human life. The heart is also the home of our human emotions. From the heart comes love, courage, fear and hate. A heart can be happy, broken, aching, pure, light or heavy. We have open hearts, wild hearts, closed hearts, brave hearts. The heart nourishes the body physically and emotionally.

The ribs should be healed within 4-6 weeks after surgery. Healing is not easy but, for me, it was quicker than most. My age may have played a part or my positive thinking. When you are 18 years old, you have a lot of high-energy things to live for, like prom and graduation. I didn't want to miss any of that.

I started to feel better physically and mentally within just 2 weeks. After surgery, I had been let out of intensive care in less than 24 hours. I was up walking quickly as well. I even met a guy at the hospital. He was my age having heart surgery as well. He was an attractive football player, and I remember our moms exchanging photos of "what we really looked like." So funny!

When you're having surgery, you don't look your best and who cares? Unless you're running into a potential mate!

I was home before I knew it. The house I grew up in has a few floors. My room happened to be at the top, so my recovery room was our den. It was perfect. It was a Zen healing place. The cozy fireplace and decor provided an excellent atmosphere that was completely Zen. The den is a nice space and also includes a full bathroom. Other than needing food brought to me, I was all set.

I remember having difficulty sleeping for two weeks. I was unable to find a comfortable position and I was still in pain. I had only been sent home with an over-the-counter medication to deal with the pain.

While I was healing and dreaming of a healthy future, I spent time with my family and had friends as visitors. I'll never forget seeing one of my favorite movies for the first time while I was recovering. It was a movie you might know, "My Best Friend's Wedding." I had to turn the movie off during the karaoke scene with Cameron Diaz because I could not stop laughing. Laughing was healing but physically very painful. I still believe comedy is one of the best medicines.

I had a lot of support from family and friends in my healing process. I couldn't have done it without them. My high school sweetheart, Kevin, who was dating someone else at the time, even called to check on me. That meant the world to me.

When you face your own mortality, you learn not to take things for granted. I appreciated everything and more. I was grateful for the strength of my body and my mind. I was thankful for the support and around-the-clock care of my family. I was thankful for my friends who took the time to visit and call to check on me and wish me well.

After surgery, the sun seemed brighter, and the flowers beamed glorious colors. Food tasted amazing and, this may sound weird, but pillows were especially soft. I would hug pillows and stuffed animals to my chest while healing. They helped physically and emotionally. My perspective was heightened and enlightened. The world was beautiful.

"You Must Go On Adventures to Find Out Where You Truly Belong."

–Sue Fitzmaurice

When I worked for World Dreams, I took advantage of the opportunity to experience all types of adventures. As mentioned earlier in the book, I was on stage with Trace Adkins singing Christmas songs during the winter holiday season.

Dream's Christmas Spectacular takes place each year at the park during the holiday season. Each night, a celebrity narrator tells the story of Jesus, with a full choir and a full orchestra. The magic of the season brings hope and joy to all those watching and participating in the show.

When I found out I could be part of the choir I just had to get in. It was not easy. Remember, there are 70,000 of us and they even let retirees into the choir. Back in my day, you registered through a computer system. It was almost like a lottery. Spots were difficult to secure. You had to plan ahead.

They would open the website at 8 a.m. for sign ups and all spots were taken within 12 minutes. Of course, these spots were divided up into Soprano, Alto, Tenor and Bass. Soprano spots were gone in 2 minutes and Alto took 7 minutes. I was an Alto, and in the years I participated in this race, I would sign into the computer early and refresh the page until we were allowed to submit our names and positions. If you were lucky enough to get a spot, you committed to 10 weeks of rehearsals with professional voice instructors. It was a great experience.

I was blessed to sing for four years at World Dreams Park. It was an honor. I had first signed up because Jim Caviezel was going to be a featured celebrity. Jim is best known for his starring role in "The Passion of the Christ" in 2004. I had such a crush on him from his portrayal of Edmund Dantes in the updated version of the Count of Monte Cristo released in 2002.

I let everyone know at the Nautical Resort that I needed to be notified if he were to visit our restaurant. I was home with my fiancé David - this had to be late November or early December 2005. I received a phone call from my girls, both named Emily, who worked at the Nautical Resort with me. Jim Caviezel had just entered the restaurant!

I grabbed my DVD of "The Count of Monte Cristo" (the Jim Caviezel version). David was a fairly good sport. He was seriously a little jealous but drove me down to the resort's restaurant anyway. The girls gave me an up-to-date play by play. "He is on his salad," they would text. "Hurry, he is on dessert." When we arrived, Jim had just left the restaurant. This did not stop me.

My friend Emily, who was in the Dreams College Program, accompanied me as we searched for him. We actually found him! He was even by himself! He was outside the bathroom in the hallway by the steakhouse and lounge, while his wife and kids were in the ladies' room. It was time to make our move. Even though I was in regular clothes, I was still in fear that I would lose my job asking him for an autograph.

This is when I begged Emily to take the DVD and the sharpie (yes, I had even brought a sharpie). "Please go ask him for his autograph," I begged. As a college program student, Emily had less of a chance getting fired. I was scared but determined to get this man's autograph. We were so close.

With the bravery I lacked, Emily approached him with DVD and sharpie in hand. "Um, Mr. Cavizel," she started. "May I have you sign this DVD, and can you make it out to my friend Kathleen?" She was amazing. He did it! He took the DVD and autographed it, "Kathleen, Best Wishes, Jim Caviezel." I was in the hallway with them, but I was hanging back a little. I was so nervous.

He did not seem happy, yet he complied with grace. It must have struck him obviously that his location was not kept private, and he had been followed. I don't know what gave it away. Maybe it was the prepared DVD and sharpie. I stalked Jim Caviezel, my crush. I am proud of this to this day. You only live once. Thank you, Mr. Caviezel, for being so gracious.

Trace Adkins is also a crush of mine. To me, he is the definition of a man. Trace Adkins is an award-winning country singer, author and an actor. He is 6′ 6″ with broad shoulders and a thin waist. He has the perfect shape, cut like a V, and it is obvious that he must have his entire wardrobe altered. He is handsome and rugged yet neatly kept. He calls himself a "free-thinking roughneck." You may have seen him on celebrity apprentice. I purposely signed up to sing with him as well.

One thing about the celebrities performing at the Christmas Spectacular is that most of them are very nice. Most make an effort to meet the choir backstage before the performance. Trace Adkins was one such celebrity. We were all backstage and he came out of his dressing room just to say hi. I was not very close to him, so I waved. He waved back at me. He was humble. I was smitten.

Susan Lucci was also an honor to perform with. She is best known for her portrayal of Erica Kane on the late ABC daytime drama "All My Children." It took 19 straight years of nominations but she finally won the best actress category at the Daytime Emmys for her work as Erica Kane on "All My Children" - another humble celebrity.

Susan stands at about 5′ and may weigh 95-100 lbs. She is even more beautiful in person and carries herself gracefully. She is kind and polite, and although I did not interact with her then, I would interact with her at the Nautical Resort later in the year, while she was in town again. I did not stalk her though!

We used to have something called Exclusive Daytime TV Stars Weekend at World Dreams Park. This was when the biggest stars of the daytime soap operas visited the park for special shows and meet-and-greets. Being a team member, I was able to attend this event for free. Something else happened though.

I was still working at the Nautical Resort during this event. To my surprise, the actors were staying at our resort! When I came into work it was like Pine Valley (the made up town from "All My Children") and I was in heaven. It was surreal. I met and saw everyone. What a pleasure. What a gift! This girl (me) was in her Zen for sure.

Susan frequented our restaurant and humbly was given a private space to enjoy her company and their meals without disturbance. Our oldest, most seasoned server was Jackie. Jackie was the only one allowed to wait on her. Just as I did with Jim, my fondness of Susan was known throughout the restaurant. Jackie was so good to me! She handed me things to take to her table like a beverage. I was in awe of Susan's beauty and grace. She was very nice and very humble. She was dining with a smaller group that included her husband. When I approached the table, I was greeted with a smile and I said hello to her. She was kind to me, and it was a pleasure meeting her.

Some celebs were a different story. There was a female celebrity that wasn't very nice. She is known as a diva behind the scenes at Dreams, which is unfortunate. Before her visits to World Dreams Resorts during the time I worked there, I had been a fan. Her acting is incredible, and I had enjoyed her work. Occasionally, I'll still watch her on her popular daytime talk TV show. It is entertaining. The other ladies on the show are lovely.

When I was working at Dream's Hawaiian Resort, we had cleared the entire building of the private suites and reserved it for her. I was excited to meet her. I was working in private dining at the time (room service). She was due to stay with us for almost a week.

I was not going to be the room service attendant. Everyone knew she had me starstruck. Just like with Susan Lucci, she would be taken care of by the oldest team member with the most seniority. This was my friend Dino. I knew I would be accompanying him to the room at some point just to meet her. Again, this was a nice gesture from Dino to allow me to tag along in hopes to meet her, even though he was pretty sure her assistant would be the one to greet us at the door.

The disappointment came the day of her check in when, with no notice to us at The Hawaiian, she had moved over to the Magnificent Dreams Resort. We had blocked the suites for her and with no occupancy there, it not only affected my hopes of meeting her but my finances as well. Speaking about this with other team members, I learned several similar scenarios where she had played diva all over World Dreams.

I will share two stories with you. Allegedly, she was at a restaurant at Dream's Lion's Den Resort. She was sitting in the private wine room, which had glass walls you could see through. Instead of being comfortable and choosing a different seat, she proceeded to sit where she could face the guests in the restaurant, and everyone could view her. She complained of being in an aquarium-like section where she was not given privacy because all the patrons were staring at her.

Speaking of aquariums, the other story I have for you revolves around one. The Aqua Aquarium at World Dreams Park is a unique dining experience. Amazing doesn't begin to describe the ambiance. Not only is the food great, featuring gourmet seafood, but the front wall is a live aquarium where you can see exotic sea animals, beautiful fish and sharks. It is a great experience if you get to eat there. It is a bit pricey, but the value is worth every penny.

So according to the alleged story I heard, this said celebrity entered with her entourage of approximately 12 people. They were set up to sit by the front of the aquarium and instead of coming in quietly, she made a scene. There was apparently a situation about who was going to sit where. The 12 of them, including this said celebrity, were standing and discussing where everyone was to sit. Apparently, this went on for a moment, attracting attention.

Of course, she attracted the same attention anyone would. People had noticed it was her and again she was upset that she was recognized. To this, all I can say is, don't make a scene in any restaurant no matter who you are if you don't want spectators.

After what she did at the Hawaiian and the stories I heard from countless team members, believing each one, I am not a fan anymore. She may not care that I am not a fan, but I am seriously disappointed. Don't you remember where you came from or the advantages you have? Like they say, it costs nothing to be nice. You never know who is watching.

Enough with her, let's move on to my biggest disappointment: "said male celebrity." He is an actor and comedian. I was such a fan watching his shows and reading his book. Coming from humble beginnings, you would expect more. In the late 1980s, said celebrity was homeless for three years. When not performing gigs, he slept in his car and used gas stations to shower and clean up in.

I was working at a buffet restaurant at The Lion's Den Resort. Said celebrity was in town for an event. He came into our restaurant, a

BUFFET. He had an entourage. They took a large table off to the side. He proceeded to go to the breakfast buffet by himself. He did not ask his waitress or anyone in his entourage to get his own food. Humble, right? No!

He began to complain to the management almost immediately that his dining experience was negative because of all the unwanted attention he was getting. He made the management open the closed restaurant next door. This other restaurant was only open for dinner and he had come in for breakfast.

He and his entourage were given the whole restaurant with a private server. Food from the buffet was brought in. He continued to use the restaurant like that during the rest of his visit. I was so disappointed in his diva behavior. Why go to a buffet? Why not just send someone to get your food and stay at your table where you wouldn't be disturbed? He could have ordered room service and avoided people all together.

I was a fan and this disappointed me. The people bothering you at the buffet are the same people that made you rich, famous and gave you a home. Even after all this, I occasionally watch his game show where families compete together for prizes, but I still think he is fake. It is sad that a man that came from humble beginnings could forget that so quickly.

"When I wear Pink I feel like a Zen Garden."
–Unknown

Working at World Dreams brought me a lot of Zen, especially when I was able to step outside my role and sometimes my comfort zone as well. I was blessed to work a lot of exclusive events. Being a server, I was able to work catering events, but my adventures didn't stop there.

I loved working conventions. At most of the conventions, I worked in catering. I was a server, so this consisted of setting the tables in the room, delivering the food and cleaning up. It was important that we delivered the food with precise timing in order to not interrupt the client's event, like speeches on stage, etc. Some of the convention halls I worked in were at the Cali Beach resort, the Nautical and Ocean resorts, Magnificent Dreams resort, etc.

At the Magnificent Dreams, I worked one of the most beautiful wedding receptions I have ever seen. It was held outdoors in the back of the resort facing World Dreams Park. The weather was perfect, which added to the atmosphere. The flowers and other decor featured brilliant colors. It was summer. Everything was so alive and so fresh. The newlywed couple was smitten with each other and the guests were impressed with the venue.

There was an open bar featuring everything from fancy cocktails to beer. Dinner was served and the guests watched the World Dreams Park Fireworks during dessert. The music from the show was played by the DJ and matched perfect with the lights in the sky. We were able to watch this show with the guests as well. It was spectacular.

Another memorable event was at the Cali Beach resort. This was the ACF Grand Ball. The American Culinary Federation brought in the top chefs from around the nation. Awards and speeches were given on an elaborate stage and videos were displayed on big screens. The food was top notch, and we were able to eat the same dishes later in the night when the event was finished. I remember the fish being so tasty. I tried exclusive dishes that night as us caterers dined behind the scenes.

Bars were set up inside and outside for the guests. The tables were flawless, covered in crisp, clean white linen. The chairs were spaced perfectly and, of course, the dishes and silverware placed impeccably. Nothing seemed out of place. Speakers and winners took the stage to give and accept awards. The lighting changed colors and went from low to bright, really adding to the event. This was another magical evening.

One of my favorite events to cater for was the Team Member Appreciation nights. Anyone from 10 years with the company plus was invited with a guest to attend this event. Team members from all around property in every position were honored for their service with the company.

Most years that I worked the event, the festivities took place at the park after hours. The first year I participated, I handed out champagne. Every year, the guests are greeted at each entrance by working team members like myself.

Hours before the event, at each entrance, a red carpet is rolled out for the guests to walk in on. First, they are greeted by "screaming fans." The fans, of course, are paid team member actors. One year I was a screaming fan for the event. You dressed up in your own fancy attire and stood on either side of the red carpet and as the guests arrived you literally screamed. We would yell things out like "way to go" and "congratulations." As the fans screamed at one end of the carpet on the other end, they were greeted with champagne by more working team members.

As the guests arrived while I worked the event my first year, I passed out champagne to the couples. If I saw a friend I knew who was celebrating their service, I would step out of line to congratulate them. Sometimes they would see me first and come over to me. This is a beautiful event where the celebration and attention are on the company's team members.

The Team Service night is completely catered by World Dreams. After the park is closed to guests for the night, transformation begins. The red carpet is rolled out as mentioned before and tables come up. Buffet-like food stations rise, too. One year I worked at a dessert station. My job was simple, I stood by the desserts and greeted everyone who came up to the table. When the desserts ran low, I notified the runner to go backstage and retrieve more desserts to replenish the table.

DJs on different sides of the park play different music. There is dancing and singing. Open bars are located close to the DJ booths and specialty cocktails, wine and beer are served. The Dreams TV and movie characters come out. Everyone is taking pictures. There are rooms set up for the guests to receive their statue award for the length of their service. Close to the end of the night the celebration is completed with a magical fireworks display.

I worked a lot of events in the parks as part of crowd control. I was a frequent member of the team at the park working the crowds during the fireworks. My job was fun. It was only a three-hour shift, but I met a lot of people and made some really great friends. It was also a great way to network and find out how to work media shifts for TV shows like Wheel of Fortune, the Chew and Live with Regis and Kelly.

The job is simple. We lay visible tape down on the ground to indicate where guests may and may not stand during the show. As the sun goes down, we are given large light sticks. This is to direct the people in the dim lighting before, after and during the show. Holding the light stick, I felt important. We were in charge of directing the crowd. With us, we were able to keep pathways cleared and everyone safe. Everywhere in the park is a great spot to view the fireworks. It didn't matter where I was positioned.I always enjoyed the show as much as the guests.

During the holidays, I worked crowd control at the park. There is a special show that time of year called Sleigh Ride. We wear bells and holiday hats. Again, we lay out the tape and take different positions to direct the audience.

In the middle of the park, on top of a large building, a Christmas cartoon story unfolds. Christmas music is played. There are lights, fireworks and snow. Ok, Florida foam snow.

The park is a winter wonderland, and you can feel the spirit of Christmas, hope and joy everywhere. Working this event, singing in the choir and working at the World Dreams Snow Festival always put me in the holiday mood.

You may be asking what is the World Dreams Snow Festival? The Snow Festival is a separate ticketed event during the season. They only let so many people in each night so that the exclusive event can really be special and not overcrowded for the guests.

The park is completely decorated with Christmas music, decor and snow streaming through the air. There is hot chocolate and holiday cookies. The Dreams characters are dressed in their best winter attire. There is a special parade and a special firework display unique for this event only.

During the months of September and October, an event that mirrors this one takes place at World Dreams Park as well. Happy Haunted Halloween is a private ticketed event also with limited attendance. Halloween music plays throughout the park as everyone is surrounded by pumpkins and cobwebs. The villain characters come out and greet the guests with a not-so-spooky presence.

Upon walking into the park, children and those who accompany them are ushered in to receive a bag of candy. Plenty of the attendees are in costume and it is wonderful to watch. The streets are decorated with families dressed in store bought and handmade costumes of all colors and all themes. An exclusive parade and fireworks show takes place.

"Time is non-refundable, use it with intention."
-Susan Bonaldi

I picked up any extra shifts outside my role as long as they would allow. I worked on Happy Birthday Dreams 2017 and the local college Championship Parade that same year. One time I was able to pick up a lifeguard shift at the Tropical Water Park through the computer system. I knew it was a fluke, but I also knew if I showed up they would work me.

I went to Dreams' costume department in the morning and was dressed as a lifeguard in the full bright red uniform, including the hat and the whistle. I showed up early in the afternoon. I met with the managers there just as the coordinators were about to assign me a position. I confessed that I had no lifeguard training. They were just as confused as I was that the computer system had let me take the shift. One of the managers was so worried she exclaimed, "You can't be in that uniform!"

I was taken in a company vehicle back to the costuming department. I traded my lifeguard uniform for a similar uniform in navy blue. I was made a ride attendant. My job for the day was assigned a different position called skimmer. I was given a medium-sized pool net and stood in the lazy river collecting debris. I was delighted. I was getting paid to be walking around the lazy river at Tropical Water Park on a beautiful sunny day. The other attendants were shocked that I was more than happy with this position. To me, though, it was new and a privilege to be in the water getting paid. I would have cheerfully done that position again.

When I was at Dreams, I fell in love with working media events. Some of my favorites were Wheel of Fortune, the Christmas Show and Ant and Dec. All of these experiences were great and unique. I was able to step outside my comfort zone and be hands on with production.

Ant and Dec have been in television for 30 years. They host a British TV show where their names are the title. They were the first to ever have a live TV performance at our park and guess who was there? Me! I'm so famous on YouTube! Ok, well I make several appearances in someone's video blog.

C-LO was performing and, of course, they had other special guests. The comedians took the stage while I was already in my position. The coordinators of the crowd control at the park knew me well from me working so many firework show shifts.

For some reason, they placed me in the best spot ever. I was directly behind the stage (the only one from crowd control) working directly with management and security. We were responsible for guiding the guests, horses and characters from the Ant and Dec stage to backstage in the park. I was so close to the stage that not only did Dreams team members bring me bottled water, Ant and Dec's people did too. At one point, Ant and Dec's people even came out and sprayed me down with sunscreen. I felt like I had made it in show business.

Wheel of Fortune was exciting. When I showed up, I thought I was working "The Chew." It was that time a year that The Chew often came down for their show. As a team member working media events, when you sign up, due to privacy, you are not always told what events you are working until you are sent to the costume department to get dressed.

I was excited to be working at Wheel of Fortune. What a big show! Again, I had made it to show business. I was positioned at the front of the park. Three rows of the entrance on the left-hand side were blocked off. Regular guests would enter through the right and VIP and ticketed show guests would enter through the left. I was on the left-hand side with a handful of other team members. We were dressed in professional wear and were accompanied by security.

As the guests made their way in, we were responsible for checking their credentials and accompanying them to the stage. We were given the light wands even though it was bright out. The purpose of the light wand was to hold it up in the air as a sign of VIP escort. As the guests followed me to the stage, I looked around. People noticed us.

The audience was facing the wheel and was also facing the water; it was a surreal view. I learned that there is only one wheel and they take it apart when they travel. I did not get to meet Pat or Vanna but that didn't make the experience any less special.

When I was part of the event team at The Lion's Den Park (Dream's Zoo) I had a chance to give a guided tour to ESPN's highest executives. This was so cool because the tour was led by an engineer who helped create it. There were only 2 tour guides and about 16 attendees. I, along with the other girl, was given headsets just like the attendees to listen to the engineer while we toured. We toured the magical land. We were allowed to ride along with the executives as they checked out the rides. It was another experience that I got paid for but was given the same opportunity of a VIP guest. These experiences are memories I will never forget.

Journal Prompt

What are some of your fondest experiences that still bring you Zen when you reminisce?

_____

_____

_____

_____

_____

"Keep Dancing" Pulse

Dancing is so Zen to me. Whenever we are stressed or depressed, the best thing we can do is get our body moving. Taking a walk is a go-to for me. Getting fresh air is healing. Taking deep breaths and letting them out slowly helps me calm my mind.

Sometimes you just have to dance it out. Picture Meredith and Christina from "Grey's Anatomy." They danced their stress and anxiety out. I have been known to do the same thing.

The clubs in New Jersey and New York stay open until 4 a.m. After a long day, you can enjoy a full night out dancing on the town. I always loved to go out and dance. I liked to drink too, but I never needed a drink to be the first on the dance floor. Whether it was a girls' night out or a group of us, I was always up for the dance floor.

I was a regular at Club Facade in Nanuet, New York. The dance floor was a giant fish tank. You literally danced on top of fish with only thick glass separating you from the fish. It was the place to be. It was a spot for the locals and North Jersey girls and guys. There were two rooms and two bars. It was 18-and up, 21 to drink if you didn't know the bartenders. I have many fond memories there.

When I got down to Orlando I was introduced to the local clubs and bars. Church Street in Orlando is still the place to go as it was years ago. I was also introduced to the LGBT clubs like Pulse and Parliament House. The gay clubs became my favorite because all were accepted. All shapes and sizes and colors frequented both clubs and comfortably expressed themselves. Men transformed into exquisite ladies and ladies transformed into handsome men and there was a vibrant sea of in-between. Everyone was free to be themselves. There were drag shows and skimpy clothed dancers everywhere. The eye candy was delicious. Both clubs were venues for local talent as well as celebrity guests.

I have always been a supporter of the LGBTQ community. In Orlando, I really got involved and currently stay involved in the community, aka "the family" as we call it. I march in the parades; I volunteer and attend events like our historical first legal gay marriage ceremonies back in 2015. My friend Clint had asked me to attend the ceremonies and receptions with him. Groups of same-sex couples were all married together, and local venues held mass receptions. The media was documenting everything in such a positive way. Although there were protesters, for me they were unnoticeable between all the love and rainbows.

Pulse is the club that I have frequented the most down here. That, of course, changed on June 12, 2016 for us all. Pulse was a gay bar and dance club founded in 2004 by Barbara Poma and Ron Legler. Barbara established Pulse as a tribute to her brother, John. In 1991, John died from AIDS and the club was named for "John's pulse to live on." The building still stands today, at 1912 South Orange Avenue, although it looks quite different.

It was months since I had been to Pulse. The morning of June 12, 2016 started out very normal. I woke up, checked my phone and there were text messages from gay friends saying they had not gone to Pulse the night before. The messages read like this: "I'm ok. I wasn't at Pulse last night." At first, I thought I might have missed an event. Was there a drag show I said I would be at? Was it a friend's birthday? Were a few of us just going dancing? I had yet to turn on the TV.

As part of a normal routine, I checked my Facebook next to see what was going on in the world. On my Facebook feed, friends had begun "prayers for pulse." I turned on the TV to a horror scene. This is where my second 9/11 began.

It had been Latin Night at Pulse. At 2:02 a.m., an attacker started shooting up the club. He killed 49 and injured 53. I began watching the news at 8:30 a.m. They were only reporting between 12 and 18 fatalities. I remember thinking that was huge.

Every channel was flooded with live reporters on the streets of Orange Avenue in Downtown Orlando. This was my club! For years, my friends and I had enjoyed Pulse and celebrated so many good times there. It was surreal. The pictures, the video and the Dunkin Donuts right next door. My car had been towed from that Dunkin Donuts years ago during a visit to Pulse. I was watching a live horror movie starring people I was acquainted with and a venue I had more than frequented. I had sung karaoke on stage in the black room.

Immediately, I started my phone calls. Just literally going through my phone list texting and calling everyone I could think of that might have been there. So many of my friends could have been there. When I reached Clint (one of my dearest friends) on the phone, he answered quickly and loudly, exclaiming that he was ok. I burst into tears. I couldn't even speak.The thought of losing Clint has haunted me since that night.

Clint and I would often go to Pulse together, but it was not unusual for us to leave at different times. I was usually the one to leave first. The last night we were at Pulse, we were there to attend a meet-and-greet with Chris Crocker. Chris is an American internet star. Chris and Clint hit it off and we got some great photos.

I was ready to leave early again, but this time Clint was begging me to stay. I didn't want to stay so I made my exit through the front. Once you exited, you were unable to go back in. Clint stood by the door asking me to stay. I have this vision of him staying and I leaving and it being "that" night. That was a real scenario for many who left the club early that fateful night.

I continued making my calls and texts after I spoke with Clint. I called, texted and waited for each response. Many of the conversations were similar. A friend on the other end of the line would ask me who I had spoken to and vice versa. We were all checking in. It took only four hours for me to find out, by the grace of God, that all my close friends were safe.

Of course, all my friends had not been so lucky. I knew so many people who lost people they were very close to. I had lost a few acquaintances I had met through Clint. I was mourning for those lost and for my friends that had lost loved ones.

The city was mourning, and the world began to mourn with us. It was surreal. Roads were shut down so we couldn't get to Pulse, but we were able to visit blood banks and leave flowers outside the hospital. There were vigils held at Lake Eola and the Dr. Phillips Performing Arts Center. The city gathered together as Orlando United. Strangers became friends and we would all cry and share stories together. No one was alone.

I remember being in New Jersey for 9/11. I was attending Ramapo College and living with my parents, who live just 25 minutes away from New York City. A lot of people we knew commuted into NYC and my parents and I frequented NYC for business, my heart doctor's appointments and shopping. I remembered the mourning, the gathering and the American flags. There were vigils everywhere and I attended one in the center of Ridgewood, New Jersey. The Pulse tragedy brought back memories of 9/11 for me. There was mourning, gathering, American and rainbow flags.

Many of my friends attended the funerals. Some of my friends even went to stand outside the funeral homes to protect the families from the protesters. Protesters were overpowered everywhere, and many times gave up and left the area they were trying to disturb. Orlando was strong. Orlando is strong and is united. We are bonded forever by this tragedy. Everyone knows someone affected. Many people decided to get Pulse tattoos. They are beautiful.

For months, almost a year, I would cry every time I spent time with Clint. It was a miracle he wasn't there that night. Clint was going to go to Pulse but went to Parliament House that night instead.

Clint and I would be out having a good time like at New Years, and as we were toasting champagne, I would start to cry knowing that we had come close to not having these moments. From that day on, Clint and I vowed to never leave an event separately. I love Clint so much. He has always been such a wonderful friend. I cherish our memories and can't wait to make new ones.

"Bitter or Compassionate"

You make the decision every day to be bitter or compassionate. Bitter is easy. Compassion requires us to see and care about people for who they are without judgment. Two weeks before my 17th birthday, my stepfather, aka Dad, went to rehab.

As a young girl, I really didn't know why my dad would hide vodka in the basement near his work bench. The basement is divided into two parts: the laundry side and the woodshop side, where he would create wood projects. As a nosy kid, I found his vodka at his workstation, hidden from my mom. I really didn't think too much of it.

My dad was barely 21 and entering grad school in 1966 while the draft was going on. He grew up with Marine posters hanging in his bedroom. His father had been a Marine. My dad had wanted to be a Marine. He was drafted into the Army and before they could officially enlist him, he signed up for the marines instead. He started off in Paris Island, South Carolina. The infantry training was intense. After a 5-day break to go home, he was sent to camp in California. There, they trained in jungle warfare. The training was excruciating, 14-hour days, little to eat and for their final test they took all their weapons away as they practiced basic survival being left in the wilderness to fend for their own. He practiced things such as making fires from rubbing 2 sticks together and eating berries. He had his canteen of water and had to survive nights avoiding dangerous conditions. They had 3 full days to find their way to camp and that was the final test.

From there, he went to Vietnam. He was part of the 12th Marines 1st group to go to Dongha Village. Every single day, there were battles and the enemy hit the compound every night. The men would take turns on the machine gun in 4-hour shifts. They slept in wood cots below a pipe rack that had netting to protect against the insects and critters, such as rats the size of cats, from coming in.

His tour was for 13 months but was extended. He was a Lieutenant. When his replacement arrived, the new Lieutenant lasted about 48 hours and then his head was blown off. My dad needed to stay longer for another replacement. In 1967, 300+ Marines were killed a day. The special forces Green Berets were stationed next to them and his cousin was a part of this group. He spent the night with him before he was killed. His friend Terry Leach also had his head blown off when he was just 18 years old. I asked my dad if he was scared, and he replied that you had to have the mindset of, "I'm gonna get out of this."

My dad was hit with shrapnel, and he has a big scar still from that day on his upper arm. When he was sent back to the states from Vietnam he worked at Quantico. He was part of the table of organization working on charts deciding where the troops would go. After his time there, he worked for the secretary of defense at the Pentagon. At the time, the secretary of defense was Melvin Laird and my dad traveled with him often.

All in all, my dad enjoyed the Marines. Coming back, a lot of the men had PTSD and were hospitalized. "What doesn't kill you can make you an alcoholic." -Unknown. My dad turned to drinking to calm the nightmares. He told me recently, "I don't think anyone drinks with the intention to pass out." He still had memories to deal with from Vietnam. Memories that are so painful he doesn't even share. I know he went without food and his boots were soaked with mud and water creating an unhealthy environment for his feet. He lost weight and glimpses of hope. When he was over there, he watched men die every day. There was also the scar left on his arm. When he returned home after 2 tours, he was greeted by his fiancée who told him she was leaving him for another man. I also have heard the awful stories about the troops returning home to literally be spat on by those who were against this war.

His addiction started out slow but then became an everyday thing. He was a functioning alcoholic. He could drink all night and be fully functioning for work the next day. I don't think he even knew what it was doing to his life. Thankfully, as a child, I didn't know much either. It had affected his marriage to my mother. Apparently, my mother had given him an ultimatum - it was the booze or us. Thankfully, he chose us, but it was not an easy road.

My dad left the house two weeks before my 17th birthday. He entered a rehab about 45 minutes away from us. My sister and I were given little notice of his departure and still, at 17 years old, this was very confusing.

On my 17th birthday, I had a choice to visit him for the first time or to stay home. Instead of getting my license like most kids on their 17th birthday in New Jersey, I was visiting my dad in rehab. I remember seeing him and feeling sad. It was like he was locked up and, in a way, he was because of his intensive treatment plan. He did his best to remain upbeat. I was not so upbeat. It was a strange thing being in a room so bland with my family sitting around trying to have a normal conversation. My stepfather promised me when he finished treatment that I would get proper driving lessons and we would buy a car.

This held to be true, although it would be many months from November. My dad getting treatment was a secret. This was private and not something we were allowed to talk about. I was given permission and the privilege of telling our story for this book. My hope is that someone finds hope in this story and knows that they are not alone. No matter your struggle, with the right will and why you can overcome anything. My dad is my hero.

The stigma was there with addiction. Some people don't understand it and others fear it. Through my own experience, I have seen the light at the end of the tunnel. I learned that alcoholism is a disease. I was able to begin to understand that people with this disease are a victim to the drug; the drug in this case being alcohol. With this understanding, I was able to find forgiveness instead of only judgment. My dad was making a brave choice in taking care of himself and it certainly was out of his comfort zone.

I am blessed that my dad worked and continues to work so hard on himself. Unfortunately, those who don't understand do tend to judge. My mother wanted my family to avoid the attention and the stigma. She tried to protect my sister and I. When friends came over and they asked where he was, we would simply reply, "On a business trip." No one seemed to question that. It is sad that there is still a stigma and judgment because I don't know anything braver than a man or woman willing to do whatever it takes to heal themselves.

It was months before he came home and months that we would visit him. We got into a routine where we would eat dinner at Boston Market and listen to the "Evita" soundtrack. My mother made it fun. It almost seemed normal. My dad and I would discuss books by John Grisham and homework. I could still witness the loving energy between my parents.

"Stigmatizing people who struggle with addiction certainly won't help them heal."

- Scott Stabile

Like many, my dad suffers from alcohol addiction. Those who battle addiction need and deserve kindness and compassion. All over the world, brave people are choosing to set themselves free from their addictions, and this is no easy journey.

I am proud to say he is 25 years sober today and that was not a quick and easy journey. There are many obstacles an alcoholic must endure while becoming sober. When you remove alcohol from the alcoholic, they have to deal with their feelings without masking them. I don't know about you, but I have had plenty of days and nights masking my sorrows in the company of alcohol. We all make unhealthy choices and sometimes that is to avoid pain and discomfort.

Sobriety is impossible without choice. My dad chooses every day, again and again, not to drink. He continues to find himself and heal. Working to heal our past is a chore not everyone is willing to take. With so much anger and violence in the world, it is no surprise people choose to avoid their real lives and mask the pain.

Through sobriety, my stepfather learned ways to deal with different emotions like anger. Today, he is a different man than I grew up with. My dad is very laid back and doesn't yell like he did years ago when I was a teenager. I feel like he is more loving toward my mom. They have witty banter. They also still look at each other like they are teenagers. My mother has always stood by my stepfather and he continues to stand by her.

I didn't always have a great relationship with my stepfather. Today, we are best friends, but that took time. When I was a young girl, I had a really hard time with math in school. My dad (aka stepdad) was really tough on me. He tutored me on my math homework because he wanted me to succeed. We would sit for what seemed to be hours working on my math homework. Often, I would get frustrated, but he would keep me working on a math problem until I got it right. This created a little friction in our father-daughter relationship. I was angry and resentful toward him for pushing me.

My biological father was part of my life until I was about 12 years old. I had a hard time with my parents being divorced. Like many children, I wanted my parents back together and my stepfather out of the picture. There are moments I remember of my sister and I saying to him, "You're not my dad." This really upset him to the point one time he yelled back at us saying, "No I'm not."

Whenever my stepfather raised his voice it would scare me. Loud noises always scared me. A 6' 1" marine yelling is scary. He has a deep voice and an angry face when he is upset. There are a few times I remember him drunk and yelling. It was not a happy scene. Fortunately, this was not a regular occurrence. We never talked about his alcoholism, and my sister and I really knew little about it. I had no idea the battles he was having within himself. He seemed sober most of the time; however, this is from the perception of a child.

My dad started attending counseling for his alcohol addiction when I was 17 years old. This was before my sister and I knew how serious his problem was and he would be sent to rehab. It was something he tried to keep private including from my sister and me. We would have dinner as a family and then he would go out somewhere and return a couple hours later.

One night I confronted my mother. I asked her where he was going after dinner on select nights. She did not give me a straight answer. She tried to say they were business meetings. At this point I told her he must be cheating on her. I said, "Mom, he leaves in jeans and a t-shirt. He is not going to a business meeting." This was when my mother confessed that he was going to counseling for his alcoholism. I remember thinking that was great. I smiled and hugged her. Our family was healing.

"A Sad Soul Can Kill You Quicker Than a Germ."
- John Steinbeck

I believe that when we think about healing, the first thing we think of is our bodies. The second thing we think of healing is our minds. Mental health is just as important as physical health.

With the help of some of the world's greatest doctors, nurses and hospital staff, my body began healing my heart at 5 months old. Through the years, my heart has been sick, hurt, loved and healed both physically and emotionally. To this day, I believe it was easier to heal from heart surgery than it was some of my breakups.

When I invest my time in a person, I give 100%. I have had my heart broken just like everyone else. For me, when a relationship had ended in the past, I allowed my emotions to get the best of me. I am still learning how to gracefully exit a once loving relationship.

Throughout our lives we are driven by every emotion possible. Those who are mentally healthy have learned to harness and use their emotions for their wellbeing. When you want to achieve more control over your emotions you must be open, vulnerable and honest. You have to be real with yourself and others.

We all have childhood trauma. Ok, my high school sweetheart Kevin didn't, but most people do. Then there are lessons throughout our life that can come with some pain, anger, fear, anxiety, resentment, etc. We must deal with these experiences and emotions or they will follow us. They will control us. We need to let go of the bad to attract the good.

I believe in the mind-body connection. If you are unhealthy emotionally, there is a good chance you will become unhealthy physically as well. If you are healthy emotionally, that can have a healthy impact on your body. Positive thinking and a positive attitude go a long way. Every time we are able to strengthen the control of our emotions, we move closer to healing.

We are ultimately responsible for our healing. No one can heal you alone.

You need to be an active participant and want to be healthy. It takes honesty and courage to look within ourselves and see the parts we want to fix. I do not have the answers on how to heal yourself completely. I can only offer what I have learned and what I am still learning. I am still practicing how to remain open and honest with myself while looking at what I need to heal.

We all know what it is like to feel angry, disappointed, or misunderstood. We have all been hurt by people, and we must accept that we have all hurt people too, intentional or not. Visiting the past may seem like a bad idea. I suggest visiting the past, looking at what can be corrected or learned and leaving the past behind quickly. To heal you must face your traumas from the past head on, but you can't stay there long because your power is in the present.

We can't go back in time and change things. We have all made mistakes and we still do. As we learn to understand ourselves better, we will make better decisions in our lives. We need to look at our homes, our families, our relationships, and our physical and mental health. When we become aware of our power to change things in the present, suddenly old behavior falls away. They say changed behavior is the best apology. Forgive yourself now for any mistakes you still beat yourself up for. You deserve to move forward. You deserve good things, peace and Zen in your life.

I think we need to take a moment on our journey to apologize to ourselves for not knowing better. We need to give ourselves time to process things. We may not have been brought up in a home that always ate healthy. We may not have learned the importance of financial fitness or physical exercise. We may have had many difficult relationships.

I know that my parent's divorce had an impact on me and how I get along with men in a relationship. I am still working on my abandonment issues from my biological father leaving us. I am very blessed that my mom chose a great man to marry next. My stepfather raised us with my mom and through their relationship I learned what a healthy loving relationship was.

I still experience my own difficulties in romantic relationships which just shows how our childhood drama can stay with us. I tend to push people away. I have done a lot of work in therapy and I know with every relationship I get better. I am still learning to love myself fully. I do love many parts of myself. I also have things I am working on; dislikes I am improving.

Really loving yourself takes honesty, openness, compassion, vulnerability and understanding. It is not easy work. The more you love yourself the healthier you become. When you love yourself, you can let someone else love you. You will definitely attract a better mate. If you don't love yourself, you may attract the wrong person. If you don't love yourself, you may attract someone that may not know how to love you. They say like attracts like. I don't want to attract someone that doesn't love themselves.

In the past, I attracted the wrong person more than once. The worst person for me was in 2017. When I was strong enough to leave this toxic relationship, I looked back. I wondered why I had put up with being treated so awfully. The answer was simple... I did not love myself enough. Being mistreated is not your fault; however, if you continue to allow it, it becomes so. Only you can break the cycle. You need to decide what is working and what isn't.

With self-love comes strength, growth and worth. The more I learn to love myself the more I seem to attract better people into my life. Positive attracts positive. Healthy connections are formed with healthy people. This includes friendships and business relationships, too.

There may be conflict in friendships. I haven't always agreed with my friends and I know they don't always agree with me. Sometimes my anxiety and depression get in the way of me expressing myself correctly. I am a homebody, and I have had people take it personally when I wanted to be alone.

I have found it imperative to be honest in these situations. There are times that I have gone places or did things I didn't want to do to people please. As I get older, I have learned my boundaries and how to express them with kindness. We are all given opportunities to express our boundaries. It is not selfish to put yourself first, it is healthy.

To heal we must practice forgiveness. We must forgive ourselves as well as others. Sometimes it is harder to forgive ourselves than others. We have all made mistakes. You already know we should not hold grudges this includes yourself. If you do not forgive yourselves for your mistakes you will never find peace and you will never find Zen.

When we hold on to negative emotions, they affect our bodies in negative ways. The first thing is it lowers the immune system leaving us open to sickness and disease. Of course, diet and lifestyle play apart, too. I don't know about you, but when I am in a good head space I take care of myself better. It is embarrassing to admit but when I was feeling down it was harder to take care of myself. There have been days through my depression when I did not get out of bed and did not shower.

When I am in depression I also tend to overeat, over drink and over shop. Not only that but I eat unhealthy foods. I fill up on ice cream, soda and fried foods.That is where we get the saying, "eating your feelings." It's a real thing. It is like a spiral if you don't learn to control it. We all have bad days and bad times. The important thing is that we acknowledge it so we can get a handle on it. Reach out to a trusted friend.

Once we acknowledge that we are feeling down and treating ourselves poorly we can correct it. We can change our actions and move forward in a healthy way. Take it from me, when you are not feeling well emotionally, move your body. Go for a walk, eat healthy, take a shower, read a book and try some yoga. Exercise helps boost the immune system. I use these techniques and more.

Breathing techniques and different yoga positions really target the mind and body. Another technique that is a go to for me is aromatherapy with essential oils. Aromatherapy can stimulate and invigorate. I love my diffuser. I most often use lavender oil for relaxation. You can breathe aromatherapy in with a diffuser or apply on the skin. The goal is to bring harmony and balance to the mind, body and soul.

Sometimes I find an inspirational video to watch on YouTube. What you put in your mind can heal you if it is positive. There are also great meditations that you can find on YouTube. Calming sounds and soothing music can lower stress hormones as well as produce pleasure endorphins.

Massage is a great therapy that works on relieving pain and illness. There are many types of massage, such as trigger point, deep tissue, Swedish and shiatsu. Massage frees endorphins as well as benefits the stomach, intestine and colon. Massage seems to help diabetes, migraines, anxiety and asthma. Touch is known to boost serotonin. A hug, kiss and handshake go a long way.

Life is short and we need to spend as much time happy as possible. Time is nonrefundable. Like I said, there have been times in my life where I didn't get out of bed. What a waste of time. I will never get that time back. I lost time in my life to not dealing with my emotions.

Meditation

Forgiveness meditation provides us a way to move forward. The power of this practice is that we don't have to believe it for it to work. Healing is something that our body naturally does. Give it time and be compassionate with yourself. If the memories or feelings become too much it is ok to step away for a bit. Just as with our other meditation practices, picture yourself in a healing, protective light. Repeat in your head or out loud, "I forgive you and I forgive myself."

I have been incredibly blessed to have a good support system. The other thing I have learned while being open and vulnerable is to call a trusted friend. When I admit to them that I am depressed they are eager to help. "Let's go out." "Let's go for a walk." When I call my friend Jim, he asks me to go for a bike ride. With support from my friends and family it is easier to get out of my depression.

I have a chemical imbalance. This could stem from the heart surgery, but it is not for sure. I do use medication prescribed by my doctor. I am actively involved with a psychiatrist and therapist. Years ago, I would have never talked about this let alone share it in a book. Today, I know it is important to talk about because there are a lot of people in similar situations who are getting help or need help. I want to help break the stigma.

I benefit from a team helping me with my depression. My team consists of friends, family, a psychiatrist and a therapist. I have had suicidal thoughts in the past. This was years ago. I have not had those thoughts, thankfully, for quite some time.

My dad (aka stepdad) has been one of the most influential people in my life when it has come to treating my depression. He was always the first to notice if I was over medicated or if my medication was not working. Years ago, I called him one fateful day telling him I was going to end it. I told him to say goodbye to everyone for me. I also told him I would not be talking to my psychiatrist or therapist. I had made the decision and I knew if I called them and told them it would mean that I wanted help. I told my dad the same thing.

Normally, my dad does not express his emotions, but because of the circumstances, that day was different. He talked about his challenging past from Vietnam and his family life. He also told me he loved me, which to this day he says rarely. He doesn't say it because he is not super emotional, not because he doesn't love me. It was through his patience and love that he persuaded me not to go through with ending my life. I am forever grateful that he loves me and did not give up on me.

It is still unknown whether heart disease promotes depression or vice versa. Through medical research, we know that higher levels of stress hormones are one of the physiological changes that occur when having heart disease. This is why so many heart patients suffer from anxiety and depression.

It is proven that our immune systems are affected by our emotions. This is true for everyone, not just heart patients. Depression is proven to lower our immunity against disease. Not everyone has depression because of biochemical emotions. Depression can come from emotions of loved one's death or the loss of a job. Depression can stem from loneliness. Causes of depression are still being studied all over the world.

Pain, anger, love, happiness and fear occur in the body as much as the mind. Too much anger results in depression. The same is true for unrepressed feelings. Anger has the most effect on the heart. I have struggled with this myself. There is a link between depression and illness. Destructive emotions create destruction on our bodies. I believe the spiritual goals of Zen Buddhism help to provide me with a path to spiritual harmony. The thing is there is no false hope, and anyone can come out of the darkness.

"To avoid illness, eat less. To have a long life, worry less."

-Chinese Proverb

"Forget the past.

Do Stuff.

Talk to strangers.

Stay in touch.

Stop venting and complaining.

Go Outside.

Spread joy.

Never bother with people you hate.

Don't expect it to last forever. Everything ends and that's ok.

Stop buying useless crap.

Make mistakes

Give thanks: for the ordinary and extraordinary.

Create something that wasn't there before.

Notice the color purple."

- Gretchen Rubin

Do not let the inner battle win. Being happy, even acting happy, is challenging. Depression is a serious condition. It is outside the happy and unhappy continuum. Depression is its own beast. We all now know depression can be chemical or triggered by an outside force such as divorce. Even non-depressed people are unhappy. Why? There are many reasons. Some people think that happiness is selfish. Do you know that happier people contribute more to charity? Giving is a way to express gratitude and share happiness. Some have argued that certain rights are more important than an individual's happiness, but that is silly because everyone's happiness is important. Without happiness, where is our sense of worth? Where is our Zen?

> *"Happiness takes energy and discipline."*
> *- Gretchen Rubin*

It is misguided to believe that happiness is selfish. People take the happy person for granted. It takes energy to be a positive light. It takes discipline to be unfailingly lighthearted. Keeping spirits high takes work.

Because a person is happy does not mean their behavior is effortless.

It is not easy to achieve our goals. We must not mistake our unhappy moments for unhappy periods of time. For example, you may have a bad moment but not a bad day. If it's really bad, you may have a bad day but not a bad week. The good always outweighs the bad and if we can just take a moment to make a gratitude list it will bring us back to center. You are ok. I am ok. We are going to be ok.

We lose a lot of energy being angry, lazy, hateful and fearful. Laugh out loud. Act the way you want to feel. Make decisions that further your success and happiness. Power through your fear. If you need help, just look toward a child. A child will remind you of how to live happy and carefree.

This may help you overcome phobias and overwhelming fears. Just because you are not letting fear rule you does not mean you won't feel it. You can feel your fear, acknowledge it and let it pass. Easier said than done? It is like when you want a piece of cake or ice cream and you have the self-will to choose better. You can ignore the thought of dessert completely or you can have a piece of fruit. Some days you won't be able to resist the bad habit. Go easy on yourself. Change doesn't happen overnight. It takes effort and commitment.

Make jokes, listen to others, be in the moment, and be alive. When you are anxious and defensive, that is the opposite of happiness. So, smile. Be fearless. Take a deep breath and trust the universe. Trust yourself you have made it this far. Show people loving kindness. You may get some back.

When you give out good, good comes back to you. You may call it karma but like attracts like. The more positive you give off, the more you attract. When you do good, you feel good. When you feel good, it is easier to do good. I love this... "When I do good, I feel good. When I do bad, I feel bad. That's my religion." - Abraham Lincoln

When you own your emotions and face them head on you put yourself in a position of power. When you empower yourself, others notice, and they feel empowered as well. You may never know the positive impact your bravery has on a coworker or friend. You don't have to be perfect to be brave. You just need to find a balance and not be held back by your anxiety. Fear is normal, adaptive and healthy as long as you don't let it rule your life. Plotting out a plan for your future keeping in mind what makes you happy helps create a successful future.

Get help. I cannot manage my depression and anxiety on my own. I have a therapist and a psychiatrist. I have a therapist for my "talk therapy" and a psychiatrist for my medication. I do not want to take medication, but over the years I have learned and accepted that I need medication. I have a chemical depression.

I also manage my depression with "talk therapy." My therapist is basically a life coach familiar with mental health. We work through my present-day issues as well as my past traumas. I recommend both. There is no shame in getting help. It is sad that those who feel ashamed may not get help.

Mental illness or not, we need to be a more compassionate world. People are hurting, and in 2020, we have seen and participated in a pandemic. It is time we start treating each other with dignity and respect. We need to heal the sick and comfort the lonely. We need to take care of the poor. Who's ready?

Semicolon Project

Projectsemicolon.com

I am really proud of my tattoo. I just got a second tattoo, but my first, the semicolon is my favorite. I have a semicolon tattooed on my wrist. A handful of you may know why this is so special. And if you have been thinking about getting one, I highly suggest it.

I like my tattoo because it is small and discreet. Even working at World Dreams, where we were not allowed to have tattoos "on stage," I was able to have it out in the open without most people noticing. I also like the fact that if someone sees it and knows what it is, it provides an open door for communication. Even if you know what the tattoo is about you don't have to say anything. Hopefully, you will just feel a sense of relief in knowing you are not alone.

When an author chooses not to end a sentence, he or she uses a semicolon. The author makes the decision to keep the sentence going. Project semicolon started by Amy Buel is non-profit American association known for its advocacy of mental health awareness and suicide prevention. Semicolon tattoos became a message and affirmation against suicide. It also represents those struggling with depression, addiction and other mental health issues.

I got my tattoo in 2016. I had this planned for a long time. I was inspired by projectsemicolon.com. I believe in its power and beauty. I highly suggest you Google projetsemicolon.com. The movement has to do mainly with suicide awareness. It also supports addiction, self-affliction, depression and anxiety.

I got my tattoo for several reasons but, of course, it was mainly for my personal struggle with anxiety and depression. I have known more than one person that has committed suicide. It is rarely talked about in many families. It is one of the saddest ways to die. This is because suicide is a choice; it is preventable by the person, not by any outsider like friends or family.

I cannot imagine the amount of pain you have to be in to make that decision. I would never want to feel that way. I have felt so low before. I have been on the cusp of making that decision, but I found hope. There are things and people that are too important to live for. Fight for yourself as hard as you do for everyone else. Put your mental health above all else.

"If your compassion does not include yourself then it is incomplete."

-Jack Kornfield

Just two weeks after I got my tattoo a Dreams coworker/friend committed suicide on Dreams property. I wish he had known the meaning of my tattoo and reached out to me. I will call him Ocean to respect his privacy. Ocean was a popular guy. He was good looking and funny. We worked together at an award-winning steakhouse at Dreams.

Ocean treated everyone the same, whether you were a dishwasher or his manager, he gave you positive energy. He always had high energy, worked hard and was really good at his job. Right before his death, a few of us learned that he was really hurting behind the scenes.

Ocean's son was ill and needed proper medical care. I told him if he ever needed anything, I was here for him and I know others said the same. He had a lot of friends who loved him. A group often went out after work and sometimes I would join them. Ocean was always there.

He was not alone. The internal battle within himself must have been too great.

Ocean told his friend AJ that he had met girls who were staying at World Dreams Pacific resort. AJ gave him a ride to the Dreams resort. Ocean invited AJ to come meet the girls. AJ said he was busy, but before Ocean left the car, he asked AJ a strange question. "What floor do you think you would have to be on to jump off and kill yourself?" AJ replied, "I don't know," but he also didn't question the question. Ocean was always saying things to get a rise out of people or attract attention. Ocean loved shock value. Unfortunately, the abnormal seemed normal.

According to the investigation, Ocean went up to the 14th floor and paced back and forth smoking cigarettes for about 30 minutes. It was 4 p.m. when he took a running start and leaped over the edge. There were stories about what guests and team members were doing at the time and what they may have seen, as it was 4 p.m. in the afternoon. A popular buffet restaurant located on the fourth floor of the Pacific Resort was full at the time.

Ocean was in pieces, and he was on the ground and dead on the scene. Dreams was private about this. There are no articles, and if you search the internet, you will find about two sentences. These are false sentences as well. A spokesperson said that someone had jumped, a guest, and that the Orlando Police Department would be doing the investigation. It was not a guest. It was a team member. It was Ocean and we all knew it.

Being on Dreams property, it was hard to work during this time. Ocean was one of us, and we were missing our co-worker and friend. We could not let it show. Flowers were sent to the restaurant and decorated the sound stage where our live entertainment performed.

A therapist was brought in for a day or two to comfort those suffering, but there was no real discussion about it. His close friends got the details from his family and passed them on to the rest of us. We all smiled at our guests as we pushed through the pain. We had a memorial at the restaurant where we celebrated his life. His family attended.

From this experience, I learned to keep a close watch on friends. Even if someone looks good, it doesn't hurt to check on them, especially if you hear something. There are so many resources, and no one is alone. I wish Ocean had known this. I wish that people who took their lives knew how much people cared. Just as the positive is a ripple effect, so is the negative. It's the people left behind that suffer the most.

GLITTER AND GOLD

I know that I want to live. Even on my darkest days, I know I want to live. "Got Balance?" Me.

We need a connection between our mind, body and soul. We need to be able to show the vulnerable side of ourselves. Never hesitate to be accessible and warm. Offer people eye contact and an enthusiastic tone. Don't be afraid to laugh at yourself. After all, we are human. Show the world and share your Zen. You might save a life.

> *"Every single day you need vitamin F*
> *(Family and friends)."*
>
> -Behnoush Babzani

So, what now? How about some tools for Zen that you can implement today? This section is completely dedicated to valuable healing techniques. I want to empower you to participate in your own health and wellbeing. I understand that people vary greatly in their needs and likes, so just pick what works for you. Of course, none of this is to replace what a general care physician or psychiatrist prescribes. I encourage you to start a dialogue with your physician or therapist about blending your treatments using Eastern and Western medicine. Remember that you are responsible for your healing, but you must work with a team. Your doctor is an imperative team member. There is nothing that you cannot help yourself through. You have the power. Happy healing! Now go "GET YOUR ZEN ON."

AMEN

Your higher power is a healing force. Love is advocated by many religious leaders as a major healer. I believe in love. I believe love is healing. You do not need a religion to pray. If you do have a religion, that is great, too. Prayer heals and love heals. Try having a conversation with your higher power. Ask your higher power for guidance, love, protection and healing. There is something or someone to connect with out there if you are just willing and open.

CUPUNCTURE

I have tried acupuncture and I completely recommend it. If you are scared of needles just close your eyes because you don't feel them. The emotional release I experienced through acupuncture was great. It was healing and brought a sense of calm to me. For those who don't know or are unfamiliar with this technique, acupuncture is a form of traditional Chinese medicine. Thin needles are inserted into the body. Acupuncture is often used for pain relief but can be used for a wide variety of other conditions.

AROMATHERAPY

Aromatherapy has been used for centuries. Using plant extracts to promote health and wellbeing, aromatherapy is a widely used alternative medicine. When I had my heart surgery, the gas they used was strawberry scented. This was a technique used to make me feel comfortable. Many people use scents at home to reduce stress and promote sleep. I have a diffuser in which I put lavender essential oil to help me relax or sleep. It works! As a holistic healing treatment, aromatherapy enhances physical and emotional health. I definitely recommend it, and today it is easy to find even in reputable pharmacies.

BOOKS

Never underestimate the power of a good book. Just as a movie, magazine or TV show, the escape that we receive from such distractions can be very healthy. Research shows that regular reading improves brain connectivity. Reading can aid in sleep readiness and reduce stress. It is amazing to know that reading also has the power to lower your blood pressure and heart rate. The most important thing for me is that reading is known to fight depression symptoms. I have always loved reading, and this is a simple technique I will continue to use.

BREATHING

There are so many great benefits to breathing techniques. Controlled breathing helps you relax. It lowers the harmful effects of the stress hormone cortisol on your body. It helps lower your blood pressure. PTSD patients use breathing techniques to cope with their symptoms. You can find some great guided exercises on YouTube or find a meditation class in your area to assist you. Research and look up techniques. This is a great tool that can help you anywhere during your day.

DANCING

Dancing is fun and an obvious stress relief. What you may not know is the benefits for your body are physically healing as well as emotionally. I am a big fan of Zumba and Latin Cardio dancing. Dancing improves the condition of your heart and lungs. This is important to me, but it should be important to everyone. Dancing helps with tone, strength and weight management. Dancing helps improve your mood and boosts cognitive performance.

DIET

Diet is something I struggle with. I still love my sweets and soda. Sometimes I would rather have a piece of cake then an apple. Especially with anxiety and depression, I know the importance of eating well. As good as things taste going down, they may not be the best for our bodies or our minds. When I eat something that makes me feel sluggish, it is easier to get into a rut. Don't be too hard on yourself we must do this through moderation. Too much salt and saturated fats in your diet can cause high blood pressure. A healthy diet can reduce your risk of heart disease by maintaining cholesterol and blood pressure levels.

The benefits of a healthy diet prove to provide physical and emotional health.

ENERGY (THERAPEUTIC TOUCH)

Therapeutic touch is a form of energy healing part of alternative medicine. Therapeutic touch is based on the belief that energy flows throughout the body. Practitioners place their hands on or over the body to bring strength and healing to different parts of the body. I have had experience with therapeutic touch. I have had Reiki performed on myself by a Reiki practitioner. Reiki is a Japanese touch therapy and clearly it is non-invasive. I do recommend researching and trying this therapy at least once. It is emotionally and can be physically healing.

EXERCISE

Exercise is beneficial for everyone. Now, if you are older and weaker, something slow and steady like a walk around the block should help lower your blood pressure and enlighten your mood. Never underestimate the power of fresh air and sunshine. If you are younger and stronger, you may have more opportunities for different exercise routines. By boosting serotonin naturally, you are doing your body well. As you know there are many benefits from exercise from weight loss to managing blood pressure. I love Zumba. Zumba is a fun dance workout done to fast-paced music and choreographed dance moves. Another class I love is called Bodyflow. Bodyflow combines yoga, Thai chi and Pilates. The class and moves are set to an enchanting soundtrack. Bodyflow works on strength and balance for the body and the soul. Every time I attend a class, my mood is elevated.

I have also lost weight by eating healthy and participating in such classes. I love yoga and strongly recommend it for everyone, of all ages. The stretches can be done at every level from beginner to expert. I use the word "expert" freely because yoga is considered a practice. There is no perfection, only progress. I have personally experienced many benefits such as balance, reduced stress and weight loss. I believe you get out what you give into the practice of yoga.

HYPNOSIS

I have never tried hypnosis. Sessions are designed by a certified hypnotherapist. Some benefits include, but are not limited to, relief from anxiety, panic attacks, sleep issues, fears and phobias. I think this is worth doing your research on.

MASSAGE

Massage techniques are often performed with the hand targeting the body's soft tissue. The masseuse may use elbows, knees, knuckles etc. to deliver relief to the parts of the body that need healing. In the United States, you must be professionally trained to deliver massage as a form of medical healing. In professional settings, you will be treated on a massage table. Benefits include stress reduction, circulation flow, lower blood pressure, etc.

MEDITATION

To meditate, you find a comfortable, quiet spot. You can set a timer. Get in a comfortable position and let the energy flow. Close your eyes. Concentrate on your breathing. Meditation is not about changing who you are. In fact, on the same level as yoga, it is just a technique that is all about practice not perfection. You don't turn off your thoughts or feelings; you simply let them pass. You bring your focus to something more positive or something you may want to manifest. When you allow your feelings and thoughts to pass without judgment you may understand them better too.

MENTAL ILLNESS

I have depression and anxiety. I proudly wear a semicolon permanently tattooed on my right wrist. Again, I ask you to look up projectsemicolon. com. There are many reasons for depression: chemical, physical, emotional, and, most recently, COVID-19. Mental illness is not just anxiety and depression. One out of 5 people suffer from mental illness, so we all know somebody that has a mental illness, whether it is a family member or a friend. We need to end the stigma so that people that are hurting can come forward and get help without judgment.

MUSIC THERAPY

Look up the American Music Therapy Association. Music therapy can be very healing. I think you can do this alone with some Enya; however, there are professionals that assist in such healing techniques. Use of music can accomplish individualized goals, whether it be anxiety or help with sleep. There is clinical and evidence-based research to prove music therapy is a true form of healing

Author's Afterword

Thank you for sharing my journey. Writing this book has been very healing for me. As of today, I am still living in Orlando, Florida, and we are still in a pandemic. Life is strange. As they say, "Truth is stranger than fiction." I was furloughed from my job at the theme park resorts in March of 2020 and, a few months later, officially laid off. This book helped me to keep busy and grounded during that trying time. I was blessed to get another job, and it is my intention to return to theme park resorts, as that is what I consider my career. Working for the parks and doing events has always been my passion, along with writing. As far as writing, I have begun a second book. I look forward to sharing more stories with you. I wish you love, happiness and, most of all, Zen. Now go "Get Your Zen On" and encourage others to do so as well!!!!!!!

Love and Blessings,

Kathleen

www.ingramcontent.com/pod-product-compliance
Lightning Source LLC
Chambersburg PA
CBHW050735030426
42336CB00012B/1582